ACUPUNCTURE
WITHOUT NEEDLES

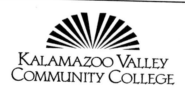

J.V. Cerney, A.B., D.M., D.P.M., D.C.

ACUPUNCTURE WITHOUT NEEDLES

Illustrations by the Author

Parker Publishing Company, Inc.

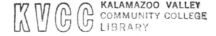

Dedicated to my daughter
Kim who has played such
a wonderful role in my
life.

20 19 18 17 16 15 14 13

Reward Edition . . . . . . September 1983

This book is a reference work based on research by
the author. The opinions expressed herein are not
necessarily those of or endorsed by the publisher.

Library of Congress Cataloging in Publication Data

Cerney, J V
    Acupuncture without needles.

    1. Acupuncture. I. Title. [DNLM: 1. Acupuncture
—Popular works. 2. Therapeutic cults—Popular works.
WB960 C415a 1974]
RM184.C4   615'.892   73-16205

Printed in the United States of America

A Word from the Author

In your hands at this moment is a key to long hidden secrets of the Orient . . . 5,000 years of Chinese wisdom and a miracle of living without hurt . . . at your fingertips, time-tested techniques for staying younger, living longer, and becoming free of pain.

How? Oriental *Acupuncture Without Needles,* and my Americanization of a fabulous therapy I call—*"Acupressure, U.S.A."* (Unlimited Self-Administration)

Have you had persistent, transient, or even local pains for which "Western Medicine" has no sensible explanation or relief? Surgery that also accomplished nothing? Have you run the gamut of doctors, clinics, and hospitals in fruitless quest for relief from pain, and gone broke doing it? Have you watched yourself age and felt trapped by time because your health has not been like it used to be? Have you felt like giving up?

Don't Give Up! There's Yet Another Door for You

Relatively new to America is a remarkable and almost unbelievable method of self-help. It's called "acupuncture," and for 50 centuries the very wonderfulness of this Oriental therapy has persisted.

In this book you will find Chinese medical secrets—in all their mystique—brought to you in a language you can understand . . . a way to help yourself . . . home-style. All of it laid out in simple A B C form. No needles! No hurt! Just your fingertips, and Nature, in its own miracle manner, will do the rest! The how-to-do-its are in this book.

J.V. Cerney, A.B., D.M., D.P.M., D.C.

What This Book Will Do for You

"I didn't believe it was possible," said John Le S. "For 20 years I had been in hospitals, clinics, and seen doctors of all kinds. I'd had operations on my nerves, fusions on my spine, more operations, and drugs enough to 'float a battleship' and I still went miserably on. Even my personality changed, and I lost my job. Then came your treatment and my health torture was gone. I slept for the first time. The tremor in my hands disappeared. For the first time I could smile again. Now I follow your *Acupressure, U.S.A.* to the letter and feel like a million."

Simply Follow the A B C's Set Out in This Book

With simplification in view, Chinese acupuncture pressure points have been laid out in this book "A B C" style. With this book in one hand and your finger on the "trigger point," you can eliminate the necessity of worrying about what comes next. In this manner, you will render yourself personalized, quality care. All you have to do is follow directions! Don't deviate! Don't improvise! Don't overtreat! When instant miracles don't happen, don't blame the Oriental system. Don't blame the book. It's more than probable that what you are doing is at fault.

Here's How the System Works

To further simplify the method of looking for answers to your daily problems, the Index and illustrations give you an *A B C Schedule of Action.* Press the "magic" buttons indicated in the treatment section of this book. Use a health-stimulating rotary motion of your thumb, as shown in Figure 2. Then put steady pressure on the same central area. The text will explain exactly what to do in conjunction with the illustrations for acupressure points.

HOW TO USE THIS BOOK

What is your health problem? Headache? Check the Index

4

under "headache" or "pain." The text to which you are directed will be accompanied by illustrations. Study each. Where *is* your head pain? Back, front, top? Look at your chart. Where does the illustration direct you to place your thumb? Back of the ear? The neck? The foot? Any other area? More than one contact suggested? If there is, then make your rotary contacts in the indicated A B C order set up for you.

What is the possible cause of your pain? Check your text. For example, under "headache," you will find I have designated many possible causes. This information was not designed to make you a physician. It is meant primarily to give you added knowledge about yourself and why pain may occur in given areas, and also why pain may be misleading because its origin may be in another body part.

What to Do When Results Do Not Take Place

To be remembered is that when results do not occur, you may have looked up the wrong name in your Index. You may have given the wrong name to your problem or even treated the wrong places. Also, to be repeated, is that *reflex* pains occurring in any one given area may have their origin in a place far removed from their external outlet.

Important Note: If acupuncture without needles therapy does not work after giving it a sincere try, consult your doctor. You will not have harmed yourself. In the very attempt of self-help, you will have done yourself a lot of psychological good.

How to Use the Magic of Acupuncture Points

In my Americanization of Chinese acupuncture, just follow the steps set up for you. Press the "buttons," as indicated in sections titled "Schedule of Action." Each Oriental pressure spot is specific for given organs or body parts. Just as penicillin is specific for a given infection or bacteria, so are these A B C's specific. For example—if you are coping with the heart, you will press the "heart" button which regulates its own system. Each "A", each "B", each "C" steps up your physiology's hidden powers, ridding you of toxic waste, revitalizing, rehabilitating, re-establishing health—and the factor to remember here is that *although the Chinese pressure points of pain remain the same in all people, they don't always operate or recuperate in the same ABC order as set out in this book.*

In turn, as you learn to control the power in this Oriental system of pain-control, you will find that painful acupuncture points will disappear under your fingertip manipulation. As the organ or system improves in health, the tenderness of the acupuncture point itself will disappear. Use this as a criterion for physical improvement. From the standpoint of determining what your problem might be—why you feel sick or uncomfortable—don't fail to use those equally amazing Chinese "Alarm Points." (See Figure 32.) They are Nature's way of notifying you of pending problems. In your hands now are Oriental secrets from the past ... and from the present as well.

TO ACCOMPLISH HEALTH OBJECTIVES
HERE'S THE TECHNIQUE TO FOLLOW

Two Easy Steps

Step One

Locate all pressure points designated on the illustrations in this book for a given health situation.

Instructions: Palpate or feel around the areas carefully with the fingertips. Mark the skin with a skin pencil or a ballpoint pen. Find each "point." Don't treat it! Now comes the big Oriental secret: *As you make contact with these "ouch areas" for the first time, make a point of noting whether pain is elicited on shallow or deep pressure. Then note whether pressure on one point causes pain to shoot somewhere else!*

This is very significant. Why? Because if pain becomes more prominent at a point removed from the "point" you just pressed, then the new point of pain is your specific. *That* is your true control point. It's your "magic button" in acupressure.

Use this amazing Oriental technique to give you this information by way of a *reflex.* It's a key to health, and what I'm providing for you here helps you open the door. It's simply up to you to use this book efficiently to help yourself to health.

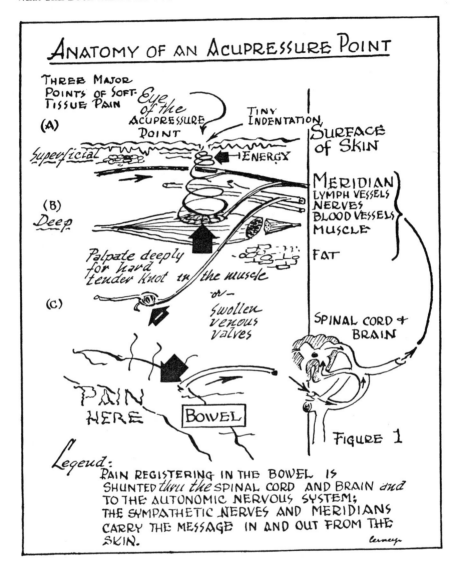

ANATOMY OF AN ACUPRESSURE POINT

THREE MAJOR
POINTS OF SOFT-
TISSUE PAIN

(A)

Superficial

Eye
of the
ACUPRESSURE
POINT

TINY
INDENTATION,

ENERGY

SURFACE
of SKIN

(B)
Deep

MERIDIAN
LYMPH VESSELS
NERVES
BLOOD VESSELS
MUSCLE

*Palpate deeply
for hard
tender knot in the muscle*

FAT

(C)

*or –
swollen
venous
valves*

SPINAL CORD +
BRAIN

PAIN
HERE

BOWEL

FIGURE 1

Legend:

PAIN REGISTERING IN THE BOWEL IS
SHUNTED *thru the* SPINAL CORD AND BRAIN *and*
TO THE AUTONOMIC NERVOUS SYSTEM;
THE SYMPATHETIC NERVES AND MERIDIANS
CARRY THE MESSAGE IN AND OUT FROM THE
SKIN.

Step Two

Instructions: Once you have located the Oriental "ouch areas," apply pressure. Pressure should be neither harsh nor hard. It must not bruise. (Pressure, when applied, should be about the same as can be applied to the eyeball without discomfort.) Use a rotary motion of the thumb or third finger. Apply until the pain diminishes or disappears.

Quite often it is not necessary to treat more than two or three major Chinese pressure points. Stick to your chart. Take each in sequence. When you fail to interpret your pressure zones properly (not on the right button), you will get no results. It's as simple as that. Merely relocate the areas of pain to rectify your error.

If pain in Oriental point "A" is gross, treat only "A" the first day! On the second day treat "B", and the third trigger point on the third day. Starting with the fourth day, you can treat all zones the same day. In other words—in the beginning—*don't overtreat! Do* give yourself daily treatments for a week until symptom free. Let Nature take its course.

Now, turn the pages and enter a whole new world of long hidden Oriental secrets. Utilize these amazing techniques tested by time. Take advantage of 5,000 years of Chinese wisdom and enjoy the miracle of living without hurt—staying younger, living longer, through *Acupuncture Without Needles* and the Americanization of a fabulous therapy I call *Acupressure, U.S.A.*

J.V. Cerney, A.B., D.M., D.P.M.

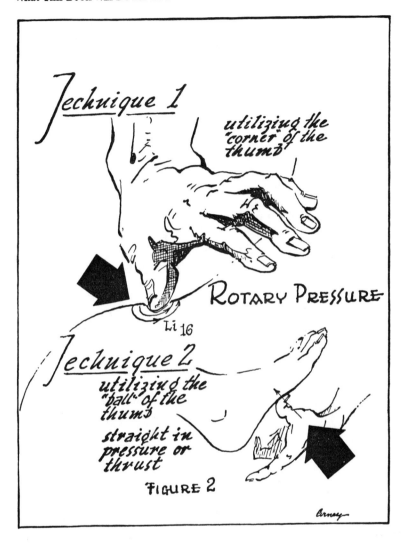

Technique 1

utilizing the "corner" of the thumb

ROTARY PRESSURE

Li 16

Technique 2

utilizing the "ball" of the thumb

straight in pressure or thrust

FIGURE 2

CONTENTS

HOW TO READ THE SYMBOLS
On the Illustrations

All symbols noted on the illustrations are abbreviations. For example: GB-14 is the 14th acupuncture point on the *Gall Bladder Meridian*. The symbols and what they stand for are as follows:—(this includes only major meridians)

Li = *Large Intestine*   K = *Kidney*
Si = *Small Intestine*   Cx or P = *Circulatory-Sex or Pericardium*
B = *Bladder*   St = *Stomach*
Tw = *Triple Warmer*   GB = *Gall Bladder*
Gv = *Governing Vessel* Cv = *Conception Vessel*
H = *Heart*   L = *Lung*
Sp = *Spleen*

HOW TO START YOUR DAY
IN BETTER HEALTH

1

My Americanization of Chinese acupuncture combines a number of Oriental methods which should be mentioned here. Traditionally, there are eight separate procedures. Each has a place. Each is applied on acupuncture positions. And to give you a better understanding of the Oriental background for *"Acupressure, U.S.A.,"* I give you both the English and Chinese equivalents.

"If we wish to understand acupuncture fully," says British acupuncturist Felix Mann, M.D., "we should try to do so in the way that the ancient Chinese did, in their own terminology, trying to think as they thought. Western-trained doctors are apt to understand everything in their own terminology—the so-called scientific method—but have a mental blockage when subjects are explained in an entirely different way."[1]

CHINESE FINGERTIP
PRESSURE TECHNIQUES

Procedure

(1) *Thumb Thrusting* (T'ui)—*"T'ui"* is done with the ball of the thumb. The most advantageous areas for its use are on the chest, abdomen, low back, and limbs. The thrust is perpendicular to the target (*P'ing-t'ui*). When done horizontally on the head or neck, it is called *Ts'e-t'ui*. *Pao-t'ui* is a back-and-forth motion of the thumb on the legs or chest. *Ch'an-t'ui* is a rotary motion with the side of the thumb and nail and is used along the ribs. This same technique may

---

[1] Mann, Felix *The Treatment of Disease by Acupuncture*, William Heinemann, Medical Books, Ltd. London, England, 1972   page ix.

also be used on the abdomen. *Tien-an* is the thrust of the very tip of the thumb into an acupuncture point and is not recommended. But don't worry about Chinese names! Just learn the technique.

(2) *Palmar Press* (An)—Although the fingertips may be used firmly or gently, the palmar press (*Ch'ang-an*) is used most often on the belly. The finger press (*Chih-an*) is used on the neck, head, legs, and low back.

(3) *Shaking (Na)*—The skin over an acupuncture point is grasped gently between the thumb and index finger and vibrated. The underlying soft tissues may or may not be involved. Individual muscles, as in the neck, may be grasped and shaken vigorously (*Yao-fa*). In *Tou-fa*, the skin on the legs is squeezed between the fingertips and moved gently back and forth. *Chin-so-na* is the act of compressing skin and muscles on the shoulders and neck. The most rigorous grasping and shaking technique is that of *Chan-Chuan-fa* in which muscles are grasped and rolled in a circular motion.

(4) *Tapping (P'o-fa)*—This procedure is done on an acupuncture point with the fist, a knuckle, a palm, or finger, and must not be used on children!

(5) *Rubbing (Mo-fa)*—This technique is a gentle back-and-forth scrubbing motion with the thumb, finger, or palm.

(6) *Two-Handed Palm Rub (Ch'a-fa)*—In just that manner it is used on the low back and legs.

(7) *Fist Rocker (Kun-fa)*—The clenched fist is rocked gently on the area.

(8) *The Pincher (Nieh-fa)*—The flesh is caught between thumb and index finger with a quick nip. Each nip follows along the course of a muscle or body part.

Over the centuries have come many techniques for using the hands in medical care. As you study the above eight procedures, you will note from such a beginning came not just my Americanized version of *acupuncture without needles* but Swedish massage, the French Do-in, the Japanese Shiatsu and Am-ma, and many other techniques that have proven themselves in many lands: *all of them working with human reflexes!* All of them dealing in the autonomic nervous system! All of them releasing tensions and bringing help to people seeking health!

I have modified Chinese *T'ui, Tien-an, Chih-an,* and *An-mo* to prevent overly exuberant treatment that may cause overstimulation. I have added the rotary motion of Japanese *Shiatsu* for sedation or diplomatic stimulation. The procedure is as follows:

TECHNIQUES YOU CAN
PUT INTO ACTION RIGHT NOW

How to Use Your Thumbs (Thumbs Down)

In *Acupressure U.S.A.*, the ball of the thumb is used on Chinese acupuncture points. The pressure is firmly down on the skin. Rotary movements may be used after the initial (*T'ui, Tien-an,* or *Chih-an*) thumb pressure or thrust has been used. Figures 2, 3, and 4 illustrate how it's done.

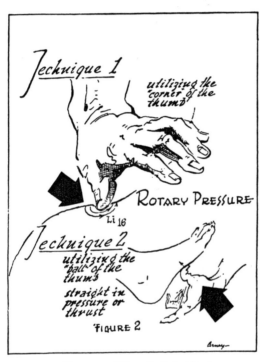

Alternate Thumb Substitute

Because some people have weak thumbs, it is advisable to use the third finger, with the thumb and index finger placed as indicated in the accompanying illustration. See Figure 5.

How to Use Six Fingertips

Index, third, and ring fingers may be used together on the abdomen and on the face. Establish fingers of both hands in a line. See Figure 6.

To Stimulate

Centripetal circles from the outside in

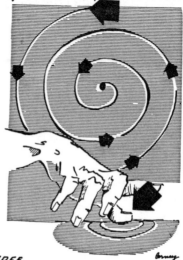

DEGREE
OF
PRESSURE:

Lightly, softly, superficially to develop "tone" in all tissues involved.

PROCEDURE:

Begin ½" outside of the central acupuncture point. Make diminishing circles toward target — center.

FIGURE 3

How to Use the Palm of the Hand

Simply make flat contact with palms down. Oscillate the hand in gentle vibrato. Pressure over the eye for example must be gently soft. It is firmly deep over the abdomen. See Figure 7.

Slapping or Rubbing Yourself
for That Vitalizing Stimulation

Although the cupped fist is often applied on the head and on

To Sedate
Concentric circles from acupuncture point out

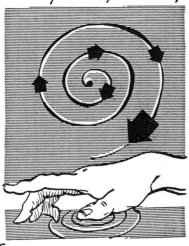

DEGREE OF PRESSURE:
Deep, slow, may sometimes be very painful in restoring flow of Ch'i, or vital energy.

PROCEDURE:
To dissipate local tension, metabolic waste, and sedate nerve supply, start on point-of-pain and make ever-widening circles.

FIGURE 4

heavy muscles, it is more advisable to use the gentler stimulation of the flat of the hand, slapping the skin to innervate the delicate but strategic *meridians* just below the surface. See Figure 8A.

How Much Pressure Is It Necessary to Use?

Proper pressures range from mild to deep and heavy. The *average pressure for sedating skin points is about the pressure you can use on your own eyeball without discomfort.* At no time should pressure violate tissues and compound pain. For stronger stimulus, the acupuncture doctor applies a needle. He may even apply an

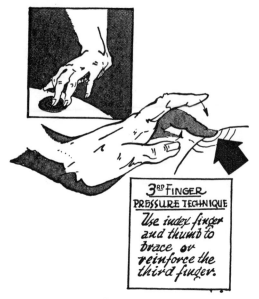

3RD FINGER PRESSURE TECHNIQUE

Use index finger and thumb to brace or reinforce the third finger.

FIGURE 5

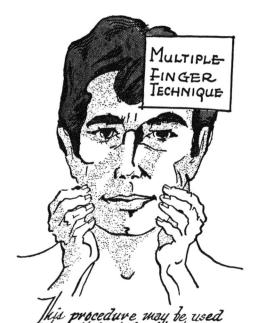

MULTIPLE FINGER TECHNIQUE

This procedure may be used where it is desirable to press more then one acupuncture point simultaneously.

FIGURE 6

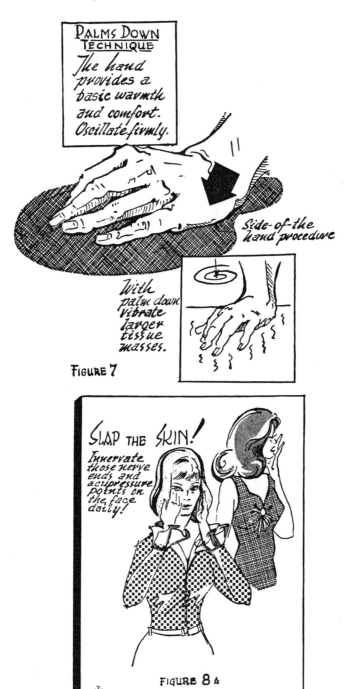

PALMS DOWN TECHNIQUE
The hand provides a basic warmth and comfort. Oscillate firmly.

Side-of-the hand procedure

With palm down vibrate larger tissue masses.

FIGURE 7

SLAP THE SKIN!
Innervate those nerve ends and acupressure points on the face daily!

FIGURE 8 A

electrical charge. He may make the needle go up and down like a
chicken pecking corn. The Japanese call this *"Jakataku."* In the
"Acupressure, U.S.A." approach, you stick strictly to the rule of
thumb.

How Long Should Each
Specific Point Be Treated?

Treatment, or pressure time, on each *point, should never exceed
seven seconds.* It should be just long enough to stimulate the
autonomic nervous system for valuable reaction and be specific
enough to do the job. *Your pre-breakfast morning check-up* on all
the acupuncture points outlined for your attention *may be handled
in less than five minutes.* This makes it a perfect health workout each
morning!

In modern defense of this old technique is the work of that
brilliant Chinese woman acupuncture researcher Chu Lien, who
states that when *an organ* is not functioning normally, it *should
receive weak, short stimuli.* This is because short, weak stimuli,
through acupuncture points, increase action in the organ due to the
influence the stimulus has on the cortex of the brain. *Strong stimuli,*
however, *act as a sedative.* The point to remember is that *when pain
exists, or an organ is overactive, the stimulus you give on an
acupuncture point must be strong!* Strong in pressure but still no
longer than seven seconds in time!

What Position Should You
Be in During Treatment?

In *"Acupressure, U.S.A."* there is no particular body position
necessary. Wherever you are—in a plane, in a train, or on a
ship—simply apply fingertips to key zones. Whether you are TWA
over Triest or in a Russian subway, simply seek out the acupuncture
point and press.

With the acupuncture doctor and his needle, it's another story.
The doctor has to have the patient appropriately positioned and the
acupuncture point readily available. Direction and angle of the
needle must be right, and the needle has to stay in position for the
proper length of time.

Whether by needle or without needle, it is interesting to note
the influence of such a stimulus on the meridians each day. It's one
of the medical marvels of the centuries and almost as old as time, yet

it's in the United States for the first time. At your fingertips, I place an organized method for seeking out health and greeting your day with a smile!

HOW TO MAKE THAT
PRE-BREAKFAST DIAGNOSIS
BY USING YOUR HEAD

Although your face may not be your fortune, it's the only one you'll ever have—and it's worth a million—because all you have to do is press the right "magic buttons" on your face to determine your current state of health. Remember, only one face per customer. So make do with what you have. Use those tattletale trigger points in your countenance that are saying in their own way, "Heads up for better living!" See Figure 8B.

The beginning of three Chinese meridians find their genesis in the face. Actually, *there are eight key meridians on each side of the face and head* that make immediately available health check-points. Figure 8B demonstrates the numbered points. Each is a key point for applying fingertip pressure in self-diagnosis or treatment and is encircled. It's an acupuncture point!

The Importance of
"Meridians" to You

"Greater attention today," says Buddhist monk Stephan Palos[2], "is paid to the interconnections between the autonomic system and the acupuncture point. As regards the various diseases, they are explained not according to meridians but according to acupuncture points." And in "*Acupressure, U.S.A.*," I don't want you to be worried about learning a lot of meridians. Certainly you should be concerned about the meridians—and learn them if you desire—but as we work with the wonderfulness of the body—your body, your head, your extremities—the grand key to starting that day with a smile is the acupuncture point! It's the button you press that gives you a natural and drugless way to better health each day. To make you more adept at this matter of starting your day with a smile, I'm going to discuss the meridians of the face and then the procedure to use on each key acupuncture point. Become specific on these points!

---

[2]Palos, Stephan *The Chinese Art of Healing,* Herder and Herder, Inc., 232 Madison Ave., N.Y. 10016, © 1972. Used with permission of Mc-Graw Hill Book Company.

FACIAL PRESSURE POINTS
to start your day
with a smile

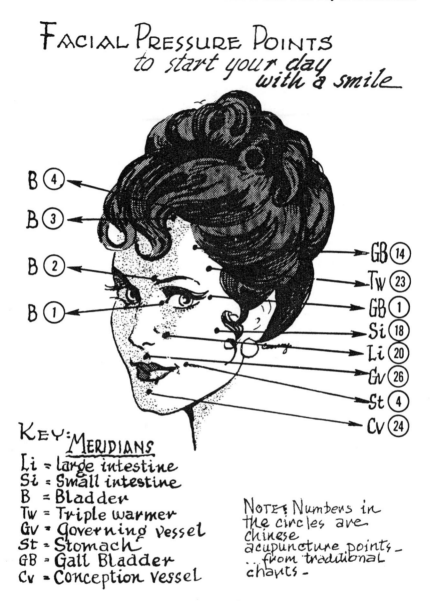

B ④
B ③
B ②
B ①

GB ⑭
Tw ㉓
GB ①
Si ⑱
Li ⑳
Gv ㉖
St ④
Cv ㉔

KEY: MERIDIANS
Li = Large intestine
Si = Small intestine
B = Bladder
Tw = Triple warmer
Gv = Governing vessel
St = Stomach
GB = Gall Bladder
Cv = Conception vessel

NOTE: Numbers in the circles are Chinese acupuncture points from traditional charts -

FIGURE 8 B

The purpose of learning this is not to develop a nation of home-style quacks with a new toy but to give you a kind of knowledge that people of the Orient have had for thousands of years—Self-Help! Self-Control! Self-Administration! Knowledge is our most valuable commodity. Use it wisely! Use it day after day!

CHINESE FACIAL CHECK-POINTS AND HOW TO USE THEM

Key Meridians Immediately Available for Treatment

Stomach Meridian—begins just below the eye. You can find it by gently running your fingertip along the bony rim below the eye. At one point you will find a tiny dip and a pinpoint of tenderness. If there is actual pain—on pressure—the Oriental physician suspects the stomach is in bad condition. As a pre-breakfast check-up warning, *it tells you to eat little or no breakfast.* When this point is painful, make a practice of using this as a warning *not to drink stimulants* (coffee, tea, alcohol, cola drinks, etc.) Also eliminate all "instant" citrus drinks.

Small Intestine Meridian—makes a loop up the side of the face, back along the upper cheek bone toward the ear. Acupuncture point 18 (as indicated in the illustration) permits you to check out the condition of the lesser bowel. If the checkpoint is tender, avoid breakfast.

Large Intestine Meridian—has its termination point just beside the wing of the nose. It is a key point demanding your attention, and on pressure will let you know exactly where it is.

Gall Bladder Meridian—begins immediately at the outside corner of the eye. Point 14 is available to your fingertip just above the eye. If your gall bladder is kicking up, these points will be tender to touch. As a cross-check, test the gall bladder Alarm Point between the ribs. Probe deeply. An ouch spot at Acupuncture point 14 will verify the problem.

Triple Warmer Meridian—ends at the outer end of the eyebrow.

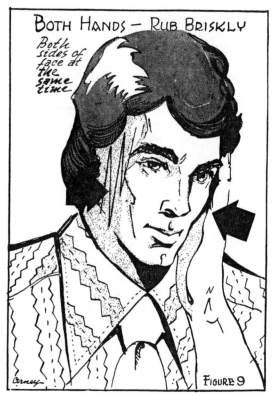

FIGURE 9

Bladder Meridian—starts at the inner corner of the eye and presents another contact point at the inner end of the eyebrow. This key area gives you a clue as to the condition of your urinary bladder.

Brain Nerve Governor Meridian—terminates under the nose, near the lip. There is another point just above it and another near the bridge of the nose. Hurt expressed at any of these points gives you an idea as to how alert your brain is going to be for the day.

Conception Vessel Meridian—ends halfway between the lower lip and the point of the chin. This meridian goes right down through the middle of the body.

HOW TO TREAT
KEY FACIAL POINTS

There *is* a way to treat facial acupuncture points by pressure. The first step is to rub your hands together briskly before touching the face. This gets the hands more sensitive to feel and palpation. Exactly what to do is noted in the procedures that follow:

Procedure for Figure 9

Rub the palms of your hands briskly up and down the side of your face with a scrubbing motion. It's a "shotgun" technique for getting pressure on all the facial meridians, and it does the job. In so doing, you stimulate acupuncture points on the Small Intestine, Stomach, Large Intestine, and Gall Bladder meridians.

Procedure for Figure 10

Now for a more specific method: (1) With the fingertips of your third finger, make tiny rotating motions at the inside corners of the eyes. (2) Repeat at the outside corners of the eye. (3) Then go below the eye (on orbital rim). (4) Then move to bridge of the nose. Squeeze! Pull! Now go below the nose to the side. (5) Make circular motions vigorously.

Procedure for Figure 11

Now plant all your fingertips in a straight line across the top of your chin and jaw. Massage the area in unison. Key points to the *Stomach meridian* are located at this point. From here, go to the side of each jaw and repeat.

Procedure for Figure 12

To stimulate the *Triple Warmer, Bladder,* and *Gall Bladder meridians,* beat a sharp tattoo on your cranium with the fingers laid out flat. Do not make a fist. This tends to jar your sensibilities. If you find it hard to awaken in the morning, use this method. Then turn your head rapidly from side to side.

Permit your mouth to drop open in this procedure. Keep your eyes looking in a direction opposite to the swing of your head. Following all procedures on the meridians of the face and head, grasp a handful of hair close to the scalp. Pull, rotate. Move it back and forth until the scalp is loose. This invigorating procedure will tune up the meridians and make you tingle all over. NOTE: as you progress with this exercising of the meridians, you will begin to feel a flush, or a warmth, coming over you. You are not having a hot flash! You are experiencing the very wonderfulness of your physiology stepping you up for action. At your fingertips, these *points* are turning on the machinery of your body.

To this now add: (a) *gum massage* with the fingertips (upper and lower jaw), (b) *eyelid pinch* with the index finger and thumb grasping the upper lashes and pulling the lid up and away from the eyeball, (c) *ear vibration* by grasping the top of each ear in thumb

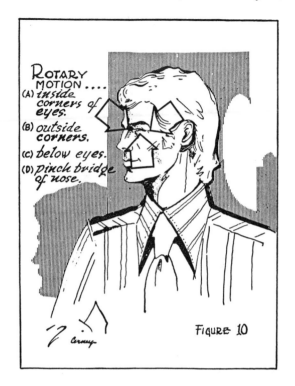

Figure 10

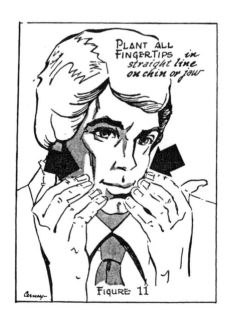

Figure 11

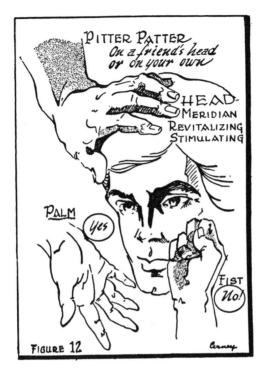

FIGURE 12

and index finger and pulling upward as if you are going to lift yourself off the ground. Now grasp the ear lobes and pull downwardly. Now bend the ear forward with the third finger, and with the tip of the index finger tap the cartilage. This stimulates the *Triple Warmer meridian* and the *Stomach* and *Gall Bladder meridians* as well. You are preparing yourself for a wonderful day with no cost involved, maximum results with minimum effort.

UPPER EXTREMITY ACUPUNCTURE POINTS YOU CAN STUMULATE TO GET THAT MILLION DOLLAR FEELING

Health ... Is in Your Hands!

At your fingertips is the ability to tune up the human system or slow it down. At your fingertips are the magic buttons that stimulate or sedate, strangely effective points that get electronic energy moving through the nervous system as well as through the meridians; a method designed to tonify the heart, the brain, the sex organs, and the organs of the belly; a method that releases locked up overagesof-energy in ailing parts and shunts it off to other parts that need energy. No one can explain *how* it works, only that it *does!* But it works, and in so doing all body parts return to health. For this reason, health *is* at your fingertips! It's in your hands, and the procedures that you follow on the extremities are simplified techniques designed to achieve health. As usual, before starting acupressure techniques, rub your hands together briskly.

How to Study Your Arms in That Pre-Breakfast Diagnosis

The upper extremities have three important meridians on the dorsum or outside of the hand and arm. Underneath, on the palmar side, there are three. Dorsally is (1) the *Triple Warmer meridian,* along with the (2) *Large Intestine meridian* and (3) *Small Intestine meridian.* The Small and Large Intestine meridians have their beginnings literally at your fingertips, as does the Triple Warmer. (See Figure 13.) The underneath side of your arm has three more meridians of note. They are (1) *Lung meridian,* (2) *Circulatory-Sex meridian,* also called Pericardium Meridian and (3) *Heart Meridian.* (See Figure 14.)

Each meridian, in being properly sedated or stimulated, is a controlling element in your personal health. Each plays a vital role! (See Figures 13 and 14 for the exact channels which these meridians follow. Note the areas where key diagnostic points are located.)

Press the key diagnostic points on the top of the wrist and the three on the inner side. Is any one of them tender to touch? Does one or more hurt exquisitely, even upon gentle touch? Do they hurt when pressed deeply? Are they without pain or tenderness? Mark the tender ones. Name them with their number. Write them down as suggested, in the back of this book, because in the future—if you ever have a similar relapse from health—all you have to do is return to your records. Cite the date, the problem (how you felt that day), and what you did to correct it.

PRE-BREAKFAST UPPER EXTREMITY CHECK-POINTS TO DETERMINE THE CONDITION OF INTESTINAL ORGANS

Key Diagnostic Points to
Check OUTSIDE the Arm and Hand
(Figure 13)

(1) *Large Intestine meridian* (LI$_5$).
(2) *Triple Warmer meridian* (TW$_4$).
(3) *Small Intestine meridian* (SI$_6$).

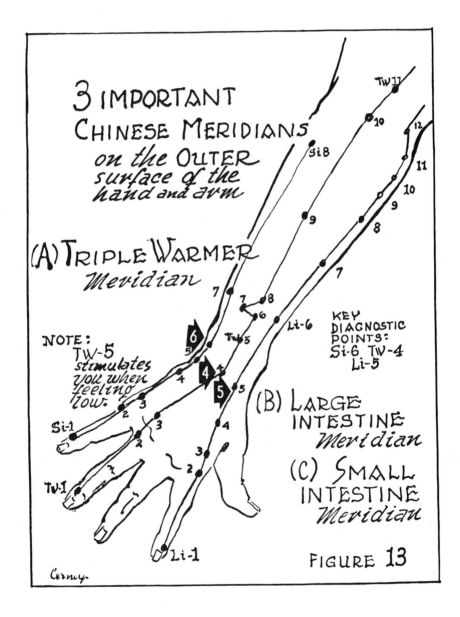

Key Diagnostic Points to
Check INSIDE the Arm and Hand
(Figure 14)

(1) *Lung meridian* (L$_9$).
(2) *Circulatory-Sex meridian* (CS$_7$).
(3) *Heart meridian* (H$_7$).

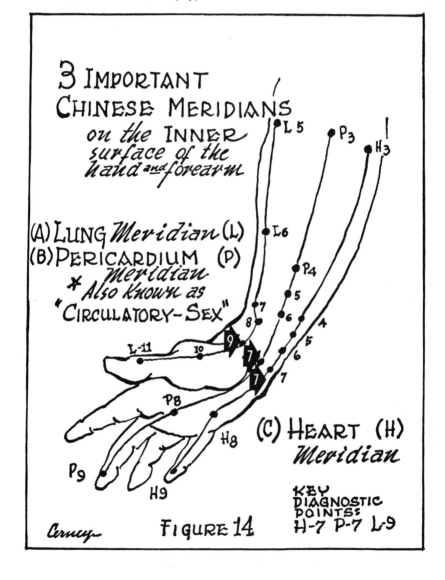

FIGURE 14

Pressure on each of these acupuncture points, superficial and deep, indicates the condition of the meridian and/or any organ or part serviced by that meridian. Now let's make some additional tests in helping you help yourself to health. The following procedures are excellent for determining the general body and extremity tone.

Test Point One: Finger Test

Procedure A for Figure 15: Place the flat of your hand against the wall, or table top. Bring your forearm up to the point where the hand is actually at right angles to the arm. If this is painless, it suggests that not only the joints of the wrist are in good condition but also the acupuncture points in this area are in good shape as well.

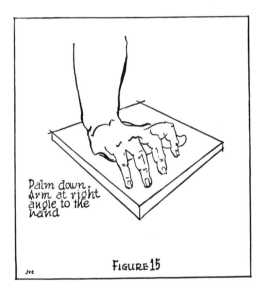

Palm down. Arm at right angle to the hand

FIGURE 15

Procedure B for Figure 16: Bend the finger palmarly at the first joint till it is parallel with the third phalanx. It may or may not make a popping sound. Purpose? Permit vital *Ch'i* energies to accumulate by temporarily stopping the flow (just as in stopping the flow of water by standing on a hose). Upon release, these energies flow through better than ever.

Procedure C for Figure 17: Bend the finger palmarly until the entire finger reaches a right angulation to the palm. (Bend fingers rapidly.) Then bend the finger dorsally. Reverse it toward the top of the hand. The joints will now show tension, but with continued workouts, they will loosen.

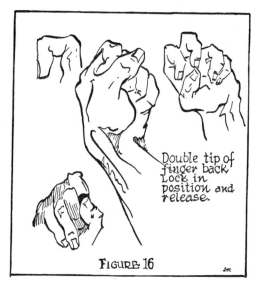

Double tip of finger back. Lock in position and release.

FIGURE 16

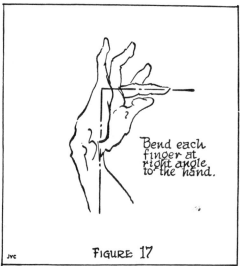

Bend each finger at right angle to the hand.

FIGURE 17

NOTE: In doing this exercise, note the joints expressing the most pain. Notate whether there are any little nodes or "bumps" beginning at the joints. Such problems on the joints indicate the meridian is in jeopardy somewhere. Notate all such facts in the back of this book. Cite the date. Write down what it looks like and feels like. This record will become your "Personal Progress Report" just like that maintained by the pro's.

Test Point Two: Heart

NOTE: The following two steps are diagnostic for conditions of the heart. Both points are important!

Procedure A for Figure 18: Pinch the small finger on either side of the fingernail. When this Chinese pressure point is tender, it tends to indicate possible cardiac overwork or distress. Remember that *in an emergency, these pressure points may be used to alleviate a heart attack!* Grab both little fingers at this point, twirl them vigorously as you squeeze. *You may* very handily *save a life!*

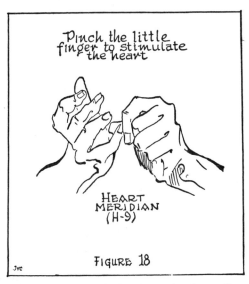

Pinch the little finger to stimulate the heart

HEART MERIDIAN (H-9)

FIGURE 18

Procedure B for Figure 19: Look at the heart line on the palm of your hand. Then, at a point on your palm behind the web of fingers four and five, make your pressure. Where heart problems exist, this area is an immediate tattletale. To help correct this problem, place your therapeutic fingertip exactly where X marks the spot in Figure 19.

Test Point Three: Lungs

Procedure for Figure 20: Pressure on the thenar process of the hand may be most revealing in checking for a possible lung problem. Rotating your fingertip on L_9 and L_{10} acupressure points on the arm, with the other pressure point on the hand, helps inspire the lungs to oxygenate as stimulus flows through the *Lung meridian.*

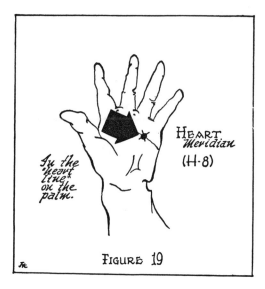

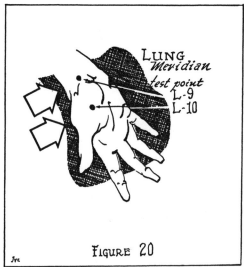

Test Point Four: Large Intestine

Procedure for Figure 21: Grasp the web of the hand between the index finger and thumb of the opposite hand. Get close to the joint. Locate a sore spot if present. Squeeze! If this spot is highly sensitive during your pre-breakfast examination you know your large intestine is not at its best. Eat, but eat lightly. Maintain pressure

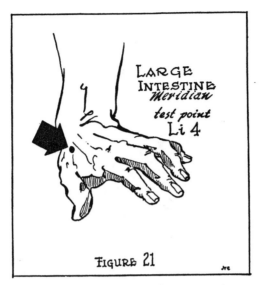

LARGE
INTESTINE
Meridian
test point
Li 4

FIGURE 21

on this acupuncture area until the hardness dissolves under your fingertips.

Test Point Five: Human Foot Reflex Points

At your fingertips once again—on the human foot—are diagnostic acupuncture treatment points that you can use day after day (Figure 22). The dorsum or top of the foot is marked by three meridians—the *Stomach, Bladder,* and *Liver meridians.* The *Spleen meridian* starts at the big toe and courses alongside the arch of each foot. Also finding its genesis in the foot is the *Kidney meridian.* It's the only meridian on the bottom of the foot and begins underneath the foot just behind the third metatarsal head. It curls up around the inner arch, courses back under the inside ankle bone, and then takes off up the leg. This fantastic network, with its key acupuncture points, is easily accessible. It's a master control board, and all you have to do is press the magic buttons to help yourself to health. You simply help yourself to better living through acupuncture and use no needles!

**How to Go About That
Pre-Breakfast Diagnosis
by Way of Foot Reflexes**

The lower extremities provide diagnostic centers you can probe

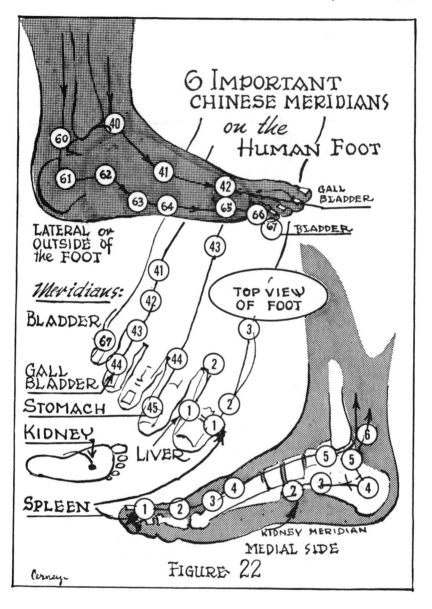

6 IMPORTANT
CHINESE MERIDIANS
on the
HUMAN FOOT

GALL BLADDER

BLADDER

LATERAL or OUTSIDE of the FOOT

TOP VIEW OF FOOT

Meridians:

BLADDER

GALL BLADDER

STOMACH

KIDNEY

LIVER

SPLEEN

KIDNEY MERIDIAN

MEDIAL SIDE

FIGURE 22

Cerney

and palpate in self-help therapy. Check the following illustration (Figure 23). Note the location of each organ or part. These reflexes are "tied" to each of these organs. Foot reflex zones *are not acupuncture points* as indicated in Oriental medical literature, but

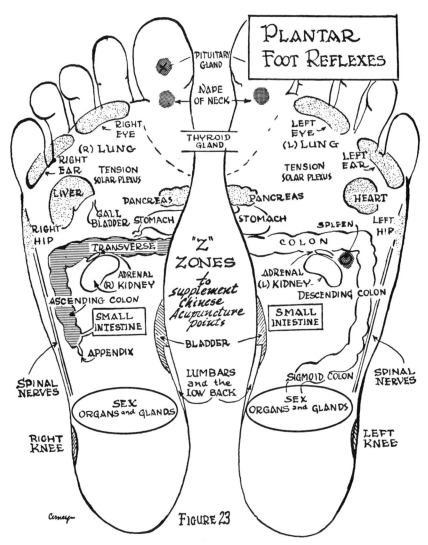

PLANTAR FOOT REFLEXES

PITUITARY GLAND

NAPE OF NECK

RIGHT EYE

THYROID GLAND

LEFT EYE

(R) LUNG

(L) LUNG

RIGHT EAR

TENSION SOLAR PLEXUS

TENSION SOLAR PLEXUS

LEFT EAR

LIVER

PANCREAS

PANCREAS

HEART

GALL BLADDER STOMACH

STOMACH

SPLEEN

LEFT HIP

RIGHT HIP

TRANSVERSE

COLON

"Z" ZONES to supplement Chinese Acupuncture points

ADRENAL (R) KIDNEY

ADRENAL (L) KIDNEY

ASCENDING COLON

DESCENDING COLON

SMALL INTESTINE

SMALL INTESTINE

APPENDIX

BLADDER

SPINAL NERVES

LUMBARS and the LOW BACK

SIGMOID COLON

SPINAL NERVES

SEX ORGANS and GLANDS

SEX ORGANS and GLANDS

RIGHT KNEE

LEFT KNEE

Cerney

FIGURE 23

like Western Medicine's "trigger points," they amount to the same thing. They are an integral part of the entire complex of interconnecting nerves, and in my Americanization of Chinese acupuncture, *Acupressure, U.S.A.* encompasses the reflexes of the human foot! A rose is a rose by any name, and pressure on these zones stimulates the organ with which it is associated.

In making your pre-breakfast diagnosis, you have only to apply fingertip pressure to determine your state of health.

Test the foregoing reflex points one by one. Then add the following procedures to stimulate high energizing powers within yourself that will step up your go-power for the day. Each of these areas plays a role in virility, capability, and enjoying that which you like most. They are activators for your better health.

Sex, Kidneys, Bladder

Foot Step One (for Figure 24): To activate the Sexual Glands, Bladder, and Kidney meridians found in the ankle and foot, grasp firmly and pinch the Achilles tendon. Any pain felt at this point means inadequate function of one or more parts of the above systems. Many women and men have extreme tenderness at this point and don't know why!

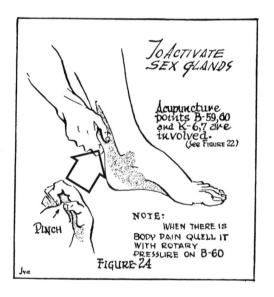

To Activate Sex Glands

Acupuncture points B-59,60 and K-6,7 are involved. (See Figure 22)

NOTE: WHEN THERE IS BODY PAIN QUELL IT WITH ROTARY PRESSURE ON B-60

PINCH

FIGURE 24

Sex Organs

Foot Step Two (for Figure 25): Cup your heel with the palm of your hand. In this position, bury your fingers (tips) in the tissue. Probe deeply. Pain here indicates malfunction of the sex glands. In turn, pressure at this point will activate sex organs. It will also relieve backache and plays a role in relieving stiff knees.

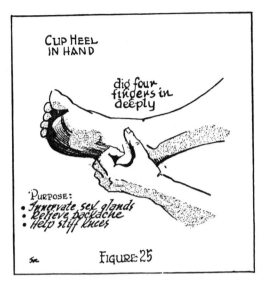

CUP HEEL
IN HAND

dig four
fingers in
deeply

Purpose:
• *Innervate sex glands*
• *Relieve backache*
• *Help stiff knees*

FIGURE 25

General Stimulation

Foot Step Three (for Figure 26): As with the hand, bend each toe downward and upward rapidly. This stimulates the meridians beginning or ending in the toes.

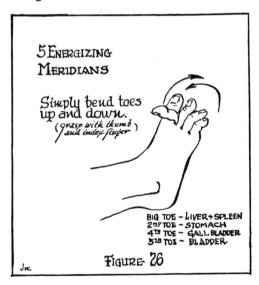

5 ENERGIZING
MERIDIANS

Simply bend toes
up and down.
(grasp with thumb
and index finger)

BIG TOE – LIVER+SPLEEN
2ⁿᵈ TOE – STOMACH
4ᵗʰ TOE – GALL BLADDER
5ᵗʰ TOE – BLADDER

FIGURE 26

Liver Meridian

Foot Step Four (for Figure 27): Deep pressure on the dorsum of the right foot—in the intermetatarsal space—just behind the metatarsal heads—if eliciting discomfort, suggests possible liver malfunction. Hepatic action can be stepped up by stimulating this area. (See next illustration for an additional stimulation area, Figure 28.)

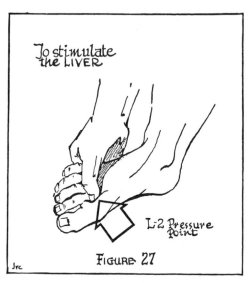

To stimulate the LIVER

L-2 Pressure Point

FIGURE 27

Spleen and Liver Meridians

Foot Step Five (for Figure 28): To stimulate the spleen and liver, pinch the sides of the big toe of both feet. The *Splenic meridian* begins on the medial aspect of the big toe. The *Liver meridian* begins on the lateral side. Squeezing the big toe stimulates both meridians simultaneously.

Kidney Meridian

Foot Step Six (for Figure 29): Check your chart for the exact position of the kidney reflex. It's the same position for both right and left feet. Apply your thumb as directed. The *Kidney meridian* is the *only* meridian on the bottom of the foot.

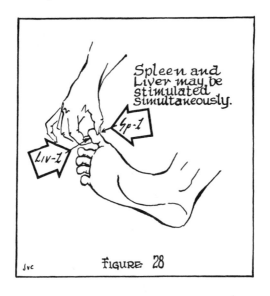

Spleen and Liver may be stimulated Simultaneously.

Sp-1

Liv-1

FIGURE 28

JVC

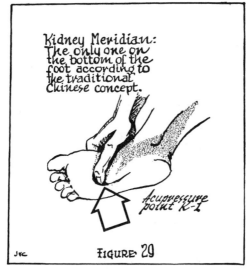

Kidney Meridian: The only one on the bottom of the foot according to the traditional Chinese concept.

Acupressure point K-1

FIGURE 29

JVC

Additional Foot Reflexes

For relief of sinus and eye complaints, see Figure 30.
Grasp the toes and manipulate them up and down to benefit the

general reflexes. Slap the bottoms of the feet for *general stimulation* (see Figure 31).

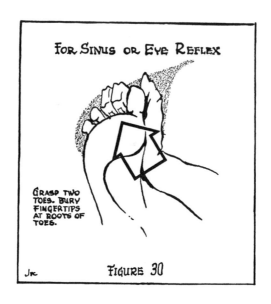

FOR SINUS OR EYE REFLEX

GRASP TWO TOES. BURY FINGERTIPS AT ROOTS OF TOES.

JRC   FIGURE 30

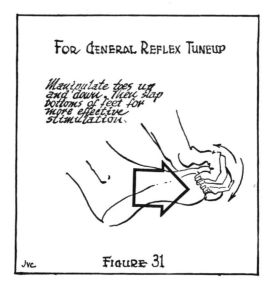

FOR GENERAL REFLEX TUNEUP

Manipulate toes up and down. Then slap bottoms of feet for more effective stimulation.

JVC   FIGURE 31

SELF-STIMULATION TECHNIQUES
FOR THE
BODY BEAUTIFUL

In addition to stimulating the meridians by way of the hands, feet, and face, it is also necessary to enhance their coordinated action by stimulating the control-centers of the body beautiful.

The illustrations that follow pinpoint easily accessible areas that are at your command. These areas may be pressed, vibrated, or "cupped" with the hands in a tapping motion. Meridians to be stimulated are: (1) *Gall Bladder meridian*, (2) *Urinary Bladder meridian*, (3) *Liver meridian*, (4) *Stomach meridian*, (5) *Kidney meridian*, (6) *Conception Vessel meridian*, (7) *Spleen meridian*, (8) *Large Intestine meridian*, (9) *Lung meridian*, (10) *Small Intestine meridian*, and (11) *Heart meridian*.

Key points on these meridians have been classified by the Chinese as *Alarms*.

Chinese *Alarm Points* are reflex areas. They are semaphores that signal the story of what is going on within you. The fact that an *alarm* goes off however does not necessarily mean that the organ with which the alarm is associated is at fault. Anything along that meridian may be at fault. Other meridians which intercommunicate with it may be creating a false lead. In other words, anything that changes the meridian and its system may set off the *alarm*.

I have noted also that wherever and whenever illness actually afflicts one of the internal organs, the *alarm* button will actually show red. It may show an elevation in temperature.

There are 12 major alarm points on the chest and abdomen. To the above-listed meridians, add one more—the *Triple Warmer*. Why that name? Its derivation is obscure.

As with the testing of all other points, remember that with alarm points when light palpation elicits pain, it means that the underlying organ is in *hypoactive* state. When it takes deep palpation to bring out an expression of pain, it means the organ is *hyperactive*.

Alarm points that are painful on light palpation are in a state of Chinese *Yang* and need sedation. If painful on deep pressure, they are *Yin* and are in need of stimulation. It is important to note that *alarm points used in this manner for diagnostic purposes may also be used for treatment.*

The basic premise of acupuncture and *Acupressure, U.S.A.* is that man's health is controlled by the flow of life force through the body in a system allied to—but physically separated from—

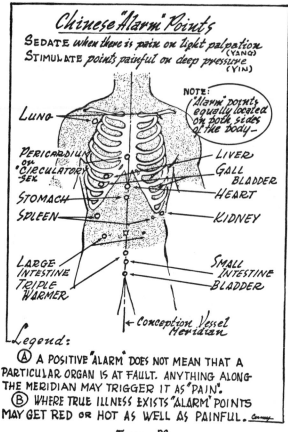

Chinese "Alarm" Points

SEDATE *when there is pain on light palpation*
(YANG)
STIMULATE *points painful on deep pressure*
(YIN)

NOTE:
"Alarm" points
equally located
on both sides
of the body—

LUNG

PERICARDIUM
or
"CIRCULATORY"
-SEX

STOMACH

SPLEEN

LIVER

GALL
BLADDER

HEART

KIDNEY

LARGE
INTESTINE
TRIPLE
WARMER

SMALL
INTESTINE

BLADDER

← *Conception Vessel
Meridian*

Legend:

Ⓐ A POSITIVE "ALARM" DOES NOT MEAN THAT A
PARTICULAR ORGAN IS AT FAULT. ANYTHING ALONG
THE MERIDIAN MAY TRIGGER IT AS "PAIN".
Ⓑ WHERE TRUE ILLNESS EXISTS "ALARM" POINTS
MAY GET RED or HOT AS WELL AS PAINFUL.

FIGURE 32

recognized neurological paths. And these can be controlled by
stimulation and sedation, as with an acupuncture needle or with
pressure!

In *Acupressure, U.S.A.*, use your alarm points as part of your
pre-breakfast routine to determine your state of health. Check each
key. Check on light palpation. Check on deep palpation. Record in
the back of this book your exact findings. Don't forget the date. Add
the time of day or night. Note the changes that take place after
therapy. See Figure 32 for these alarm points.

TECHNIQUE TO USE IN
YOUR PRE-BREAKFAST CHECK-UP
OF THE ALARM POINTS

Position in bed: On your back, relaxed upon awakening.
Hands: Uncovered and cool so that they will be sensitive to temperature changes on all body parts examined.

What You Should Expect

Normal skin: This is firm in texture. It is elastic, slightly moist, and resilient on pressure. Skin over alarm points may be pink, hot, cold, indented, raised, or normal in color or temperature, but may express pain on light or heavy pressure.

The Key Repeated

Light pressure, eliciting pain, indicates deficiency in the corresponding organ or associated parts.

Deep pressure, eliciting pain, means an overactive organ or some involvement of associated parts.

NOTE: *No pain on any kind of pressure tends to indicate health! In just this way then do meridians and skin points reflect health and disease.*

Here's Another Test
for Your Check-Up

Temperature variables in the skin: Cool skin over a "point" or meridian indicates an inadequacy or deficiency in that meridian or its associated parts.

Hot areas: Indicate current or pending illness in an organ or parts associated with the meridian being examined.

Special Note on
Elevated Skin Temperatures

There are certain temperature changes in the body of which to be aware—changes that are normal in human physiology—and are remarkable to the meridian involved as well as to the time of day.

Energy moves through the body night and day. Each 24 hours it is involved in cycles of waves of warmth. All astute acupuncture students quickly note temperature changes characteristic of each meridian. To demonstrate the maximum flow of these cycles, I have prepared the following chart:

Around-the-Clock HUMAN-HEAT-CYCLE					
Time:	3-5 a.m.	5-7 a.m.	7-9 a.m.	9-11 a.m.	11 a.m. to 1 p.m.	1-3 p.m.
Meridian:	Lungs	Large Int.	Stomach	Spleen	Heart	Small Int.
Time:	3-5 p.m.	5-7 p.m.	7-9 p.m.	9-11 p.m.	11 p.m. to 1 a.m.	1-3 a.m.
Meridian:	Bladder	Kidney	Cir.-Sex	Triple Warmer	Gall Bladder	Liver

These waves of heat are not always perceptible to the unknowledgeable person, and they may go by unnoticed. To the sensitive person, they must be felt all over the body, head, or extremities. Some just experience a flush in the face. It may be felt as a mild fever with an actual oral temperature rise, which can be misleading to those who go around with a thermometer in their mouth all the time.

The Case of Mrs. H.

I recall one of my patients who had just surgically had her bladder "tied up." Mrs. Mary H. complained of feeling hot every late afternoon. She asked her physician about the matter. He said it was a post-surgical infection and gave her penicillin. However, if you will check the previous chart, you will note that late afternoon is the normal heat cycle period for the bladder. The surgery just emphasized its intensity. Mrs. H's physician was simply not aware of what the Chinese have known for centuries. After acupuncture and acupressure procedures, her pain went away. There was no longer any necessity to be loaded with narcotics.

"Doctor," she said, "you taught me how to start my day with a smile . . . Acupressure, U.S.A. style."

HOW "ACUPRESSURE, U.S.A." BEGAN

With the years has come a refinement in acupuncture techniques, and I have used many approaches to Chinese "points" other than with a needle. Although the needle technique still persists in traditional procedure, there are more sophisticated ways in use for people who cannot stand the thought, or the sight, or the sensation of a steel point entering their hide. For patients who wanted a method of home therapy, I developed my Americanized acupuncture pressure-point procedure and dubbed it *"Acupressure, U.S.A."* (Unlimited Self-Administration).

As a remedial method, *Acupressure, U.S.A.* has proven itself along with other acupuncture alternatives, such as ethyl chloride spray, ice rubs, ultrasonics, percussion, oscillating vibrators, laser beams, "cupping," slow sinusoidal electric currents, galvanism, and a dozen other modalities, each with one purpose in view—*Get rid of hurt! Alleviate pain!*

All such treatment techniques are designed to penetrate "pressure points." They are meant to short-circuit jambed physiological systems and return them to normalcy through an adjustment of the autonomic nervous system. When acupuncture points are penetrated, here's what happens.

HOW "ACUPRESSURE, U.S.A." WORKS

Acupuncture (by any method or in any form) . . .

(1) *Breaks the reflex arc* between the pressure point just under the skin and the organs with which it communicates. It re-arranges those forces which the Orientals called *yin* and *yang*, forces that jamb channels of *ching-lo* and contribute to the illness of an organ or part. Through acupressure stimulation or sedation of the autonomic nervous system, normalcy is achieved.

(2) *Acupressure steps up the arterial supply.*

(3) *It stimulates endocrine gland function.*

(4) *It stimulates lymph and venous drainage.*

(5) *It releases waste products from the musculature and other organs.*

(6) *It helps achieve mental relaxation* as well as physiological peace.

(7) *It reduces hurt.*

MORE EXAMPLES OF BENEFITS POSSIBLE WITH ACUPRESSURE

In the "Pain Clinic" of State University in Seattle, a Chinese physician by the name of Mifoo Hsu is doing work in pain relief. On

March 28, 1972, the National Broadcasting Company had its television crew on the spot to witness Dr. Hsu's method of acupuncture in helping a woman who had received all the orthodox medical treatments and went on suffering. As Dr. Hsu's competent hands went to work, on the television screen, the world witnessed her loss of facial pain. A miracle? Not at all! It was acupuncture know-how and on-the-scene facts which can no longer be denied.

A leading American journalist told the world his experience in China when he experienced a Western-style operation with anesthesia and then had to resort to acupuncture to be relieved of post-operative pain.

A famous columnist reported how an opera star was cured of severe back trouble by a practitioner in Rome. She suffered for ten years, and 11 medical doctors told her that her only answer to backache was surgery. After acupuncture therapy, she *ran* about the room. Her backache was gone!

In her autobiography *Office Hours: Day and Night*, Dr. Janet Travell cites how she compared notes with a visiting acupuncturist and found they were using the same trigger point areas. It was this initial work with acupuncture that led her to more extensive study of Chinese techniques and acupuncture on the chronically ailing back of former American President John F. Kennedy.

In an unprecedented visit to Communist China in 1972, U.S. President Richard M. Nixon and his wife Pat startled the world by opening an international door that had long been closed.

While her husband was concerned with affairs of state, Mrs. Nixon went visiting. She toured farm communes. As she walked into a farm commune clinic, she saw an elderly Chinese woman undergoing the ancient medical treatment of acupuncture. Nine silver and gold needles were stuck in her shoulder, arm, and leg. The patient nodded, smiled, and said "hello." She appeared to enjoy the occasion. Mrs. Nixon was informed that the needles were applied to nerve ends to create anesthesia and relieve pain.

This story, receiving world coverage, was instrumental in bringing greater attention to acupuncture in the U.S.A. For the first time, Americans were truly aware of a medical procedure that was 5,000 years old. The bright, new face of acupuncture was brought to light in modern American medical care, and gracious Pat Nixon was just one of those who helped open the door. How well you take advantage of this open door depends on how well you put the following information to work. From this point on, it's up to *you*!

HOME TREATMENT SECTION

2

How to Use Your "ABC Schedule of Action"—Page 49

Fatigue . . . Tension . . . Tired Feeling—How to Eliminate Them
with Acupuncture Without Needles—Page 53

Self-Help Procedures:

* * * * * * *

B E F O R E   Y O U   S T A R T ....

HOW TO USE YOUR "ABC SCHEDULE OF ACTION"

As a general reminder—the following simplified
method was developed to give you procedures for
instant self-care. All you do is follow the "Schedule
of Action." An illustration accompanies each illness
or physical problem. All home treatments are laid out
in Sections. Each deals with a portion of the
anatomy. Each shows the "magic button" to press in
Acupressure, U.S.A. Use them . . . efficiently!

Check Your "Magic Buttons"
Carefully

Press each acupuncture point as indicated. Take them in A B C order. Use the prescribed health-stimulating rotary motion and thrust. Don't expect instant miracles. If they happen, rejoice. When they don't happen, check back on yourself. Check your technique. You may have looked up the wrong reference, treated the wrong place, or treated inadequately.

Keep Your Problems Recorded

Use health record sheets for your notations. WARNING: All progress does not begin with immediate recuperation. Oddly enough —in some cases—the old cliché, "You've got to get worse before you get better," is sometimes true. Some professions call this "re-tracing." Nature appears to go backwardly toward health. However, this is merely the release of toxic waste that has been boxed up in some organ or body part. Under normal circumstances, your transition back to health will be gentle.

So press each A, each B, each C in the *Schedule of Action* with revitalization, recuperation, rejuvenation, and the re-establishing of health in view.

Beneath Your Fingertips
Will Pain Disappear

One more reminder: Since organs and body parts do not recuperate in ABC order, don't expect them to. As you learn to control the power in this Oriental system of pain control and health rehabilitation, you will find painful acupuncture points disappearing beneath your fingertips. As this reflex disappears, it is indicative that the organ with which it is associated is recuperating. Abnormal *yin* and *yang* forces affecting the Chinese meridians are being dissipated. You are on your way to recovery.

This book is intended to help the average person return to health by natural means. It was designed to show you how to ease your daily hurts and promote well-being. What this book does not do is make you a doctor! Nor does it give you the know-how—or the right—to treat people who are seriously ill. With this in mind, here are some rules to follow.
Lest you forget. . . .

Guidelines for Self-Help

(1) *DON'T* treat contagious diseases!

(2) *DON'T* treat yourself if you have stomach or duodenal ulcers, hemophilia, purpura, aneurysm, or cancer.

(3) *DON'T* use *Acupressure, U.S.A.* directly on a fractured area.

(4) *DON'T* treat yourself if you have advanced heart, kidney, liver, or lung disease.

One more time. . . .

What Is Acupressure, U.S.A.?

Acupressure, U.S.A. is the manual procedure of rotary compression and/or thrust of the fingertips into known Oriental acupuncture points, with intent to stimulate or sedate the autonomic nervous system and thereby regulate health irregularities and improve physical and mental well-being, generating euphoria.

Is Acupressure Just Temporary?

Acupressure, U.S.A. is *not* just a temporary remedy. It is a steadying and sometimes dramatic agent for stimulating and sedating Nature's own dynamic-power-centers by way of instinctive tools—man's hands—to revitalize, regenerate, and repair by way of natural cures. By diplomatic pressure on key Oriental acupuncture points do those lasting miracles of the human body begin.

What Is the Proper Hand-Pressure Technique?

Thumb and Third Finger

These fingers are the most used in *Acupressure, U.S.A.* As indicated in Figures 2 and 5 (see pages 15 and 18), they are applied firmly down, even while making tiny rotary or vibratory motions. At no time are tissues jambed or pounded in this message of diplomacy to the autonomic nervous system. Although external tissues are probed superficially and deeply, the pressure is always gently perpendicular to the acupuncture point being investigated or treated.

Index, Middle, and Ring Fingers

In the broad spectrum approach, to cover areas somewhat larger than one acupuncture point or meridian, use three fingers simultaneously as a time saver.

Palm of the Hand

Full hand acupressure application is palm down on the target with mild vibratory action. This procedure is used over the abdomen, testes, eyes, and breasts.

How Strong Should the Application Be?

Pressure varies with the depth of the pain present in an acupuncture point. If pain is elicited superficially, the treatment should be simply and lightly superficial. Where acupuncture-point pain is determined in deeper tissues, deep or heavier pressure is utilized. By superficial pressure, I mean *that amount of pressure you can comfortably stand on your eyeball.* All pressures are perpendicular to the skin target. The neck and testes are the departure from this rule. Here the application is gentle and of shorter duration.

Which Acupuncture Point Does One Treat?

Simply follow the A B C's on the illustrations that accompany each treatment segment. By following these A B C's, you will become versed in *Acupressure, U.S.A.* Then, and only then, go to auxiliary points. Use no points that are not indicated because you may actually be interfering with the treatment outlined. The rule of hand is *"treat major acupuncture points in direct relationship to whether specific pain elicited is superficial or deep."*

In your first attempts at *Acupressure, U.S.A.* procedures, use those "points" that are closest to the injury or ailing part, unless the *ABC Schedule of Action* directs you to do otherwise. In this fabulous Oriental therapy, you will be amazed to find that distant parts are immediately affected. You will be never endingly astonished—as am I—when a kidney problem, for instance, is relieved by the simple application of a fingertip to the foot, and a heart improves because of the use of *Acupressure, U.S.A.* on the hand. How and why this happens is described in this book. Your *Pre-Breakfast examination*—to determine your state of physical well-being—will take less than ten minutes as your adeptness grows.

* * * * * * * *

FATIGUE ... TENSION ... TIRED FEELING—
HOW TO ELIMINATE THEM WITH
ACUPUNCTURE WITHOUT
NEEDLES

FATIGUE
AND HOW TO GET RID OF IT

In *Acupressure, U.S.A.*, you have a secret weapon against tiredness. In this Americanized method of using Oriental acupuncture points to bring you relief from fatigue, you have an exciting and totally non-cost technique for Unlimited Self-Administration.

Why Everybody Is "Up Tight" Today

The tensions that have invaded business, as well as social and family life, are keeping everyone in a state of fatigue.

Fatigue collects. If not relieved, or shunted away, it leads to exhaustion and even to disease.

In the process of living, sleep is admittedly a requirement vital to daily physical recuperation and achievement. But it's only part of the big show. To live longer and look younger, fatigue has to be eradicated before it takes its toll.

Remember that fatigue in normal life is not normal. It comes only when boredom sets in. The person excited about his job, his health, knows no fatigue. Hard work, constant work, never wearies him. The moment boredom sets in, that's when frustration and tensions begin. That's when isomnia sets in. That's when tiredness starts. To defeat boredom, and the fatigue it precipitates, there are certain *Acupressure, U.S.A.* procedures you can use to restore full function and have the kind of energy and go-power you desire. All you have to do is awaken the dynamo within you. By touching key acupuncture points from head to foot, you energize yourself for action.

Let's start at the bottom and work up. Remember that the human foot is a foundation. The building of the body is no better than the foundation upon which it stands. Intimately related to every body part and organ are acupuncture points and meridians. Stimulating or sedating these parts from head to foot brings about better health. More energy is brought about by pressing these "magic buttons," and weariness simply disappears!

THE ORIENTAL TECHNIQUE
FOR GENERATING ENERGY

A Case History

Marlene M. was a seamstress. In the daytime she worked over a hot sewing machine. At night she moonlighted on a second job to maintain her family. With her Air Force husband shot down in Vietnam, the burden of survival was on her. The poor woman was a physical wreck. Tension and fatigue were almost wiping her out, until she learned *Acupressure, U.S.A.* and a technique that not only released her tensions but enriched her life by making her feel like a woman again. To help her with her problem, here is the technique she was taught.

The FOOT . . . Erasers of Fatigue

Technique for Figure 33

Start with thumb pressure on K-1 (the only meridian on the bottom of the foot, according to traditional Chinese medicine). Then go to the ball of the big toe and the reflex point of the pituitary gland. Grasp the big toe. Squeeze. Do the same with the other toes and repeat the process. Now go to the arch and search with your fingertips for little nodules or muscular contractions. Apply pressure. At first these areas will be amazingly tender. Persist until the pain dissipates. (Do not be harsh in treatment.)

The ANKLE . . . Erasers of Fatigue

Technique for Figure 34

Grasp the Achilles tendon. Pinch gently. Check, by palpation, for painful areas just above the inside ankle bones (between bone and tendon). Apply pressure until the distress subsides. Then check the inside and outside of the heel bones. These are reflex points for the uterus, ovaries, and testicles. Stimulate.

The LEG . . . Erasers of Fatigue

Technique for Figure 35

Move up the calf. Compress the sides with both palms. Stroke

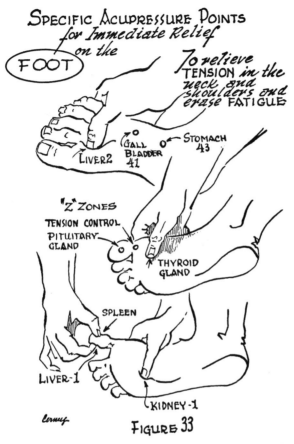

SPECIFIC ACUPRESSURE POINTS
for Immediate Relief
on the
(FOOT)

To relieve
TENSION *in the*
neck and
shoulders and
erase FATIGUE

LIVER2

GALL BLADDER 41

STOMACH 43

"Z" ZONES
TENSION CONTROL
PITUITARY GLAND

THYROID GLAND

SPLEEN

LIVER-1

KIDNEY-1

FIGURE 33

the Achilles tendon upward. You will find your fingers running over an area of tenderness. It may be shallow. It may be deep. Apply thumb pressure in accordance to its depth until pain is gone. Run your fingers up the inside and outside of the lower leg, seeking more "ouch areas." On the outside of the lower leg, below the level of the knee, is the head of the fibula. Just below and slightly in front of the head of the fibula is what the Japanese refer to as the *sanri*. This is an important vitality-stimulating zone. It's a point where weary Oriental foot travelers applied a burning ball of moxa, and with energy restored, traveled on.

The KNEE and THIGH . . . Erasers of Fatigue

Technique for Figure 36

From *sanri* (K-34) work thumb-pressure points at 1-inch levels

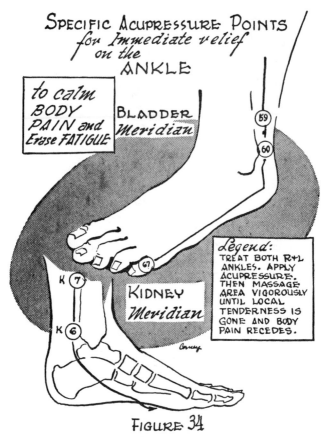

SPECIFIC ACUPRESSURE POINTS
for Immediate relief
on the
ANKLE

to calm
BODY
PAIN *and*
Erase FATIGUE

BLADDER
Meridian

59

60

Legend:
TREAT BOTH R+L
ANKLES. APPLY
ACUPRESSURE.
THEN MASSAGE
AREA VIGOROUSLY
UNTIL LOCAL
TENDERNESS IS
GONE AND BODY
PAIN RECEDES.

67

K 7

KIDNEY
Meridian

K 6

FIGURE 34

up the outside, inside, and anterior, of the knee and thigh. Repeat the process on the other extremity before making contact with the buttocks. Lie on your back if circumstance permits. Or, if you are in an office, simply prop your legs up on a desk. Now encircle the patella (knee cap) with thumb pressure points around the periphery.

The LOW BACK . . . Erasers of Fatigue

Technique for Figure 37

If this is your early morning workout—and you're in bed on your back (or if you are in an office sitting in a chair)—simply insert your fists—knuckles into the back—on either side of the lumbar vertebrae. This not only alleviates hip distress but also relieves sciatic nerve congestion. Bring your knees up. Now extend your legs. Stretch! Bring your arms up over your head. Stretch! Breathe deeply

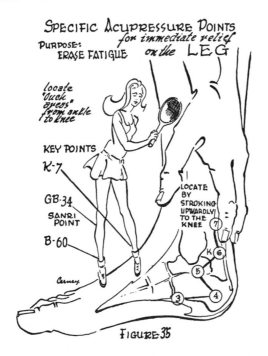

SPECIFIC ACUPRESSURE POINTS
for immediate relief
on the LEG

PURPOSE:
ERASE FATIGUE

locate "Duck areas" from ankle to knee

KEY POINTS

K-7

GB-34

SANRI POINT

B-60

LOCATE BY STROKING UPWARDLY TO THE KNEE

Carney

FIGURE 35

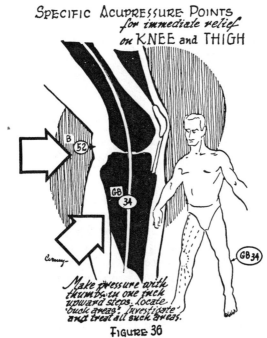

SPECIFIC ACUPRESSURE POINTS
for immediate relief
on KNEE and THIGH

B 52

GB 34

GB 34

Carney

Make pressure with thumbs, in one inch upward steps. Locate "duck areas". Investigate and treat all such areas.

FIGURE 36

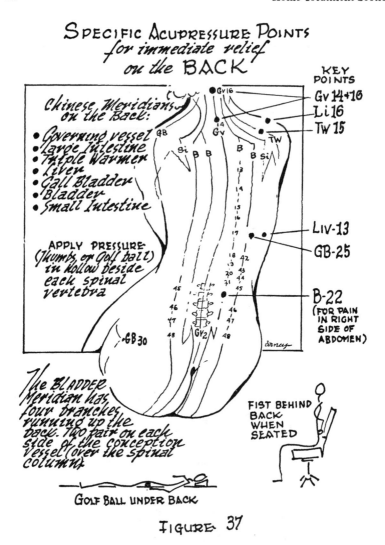

SPECIFIC ACUPRESSURE POINTS
for immediate relief
on the BACK

KEY POINTS

Chinese Meridians on the Back:
- Governing vessel
- Large Intestine
- Triple Warmer
- Liver
- Gall Bladder
- Bladder
- Small Intestine

APPLY PRESSURE (Thumbs, or Golf ball) in hollow beside each spinal vertebra

Gv 14+16
Li 16
Tw 15

Liv-13
GB-25

B-22
(FOR PAIN IN RIGHT SIDE OF ABDOMEN)

The BLADDER Meridian has four branches running up the back. Two pair on each side of the conception vessel, over the spinal column.

FIST BEHIND BACK WHEN SEATED

GOLF BALL UNDER BACK

FIGURE 37

as you are doing all this. With this initial procedure, you will begin to feel a warm sensation flushing throughout your physiognomy. Hurt areas will disappear. Tired aching hips where fatigue collects will release it. Hurt, caused by poor posture and inadequate exercise will dissipate. Potential disaster collected in the back muscles, the underlying vertebrae, and the abdominal organs, deep within, will be neutralized.

When fatigue gathers at this point, sciatica, lumbago, and sacro-iliac problems are soon to follow. So move that fatigue out! Prevent the age-makers! Insert your thumbs into the hollows

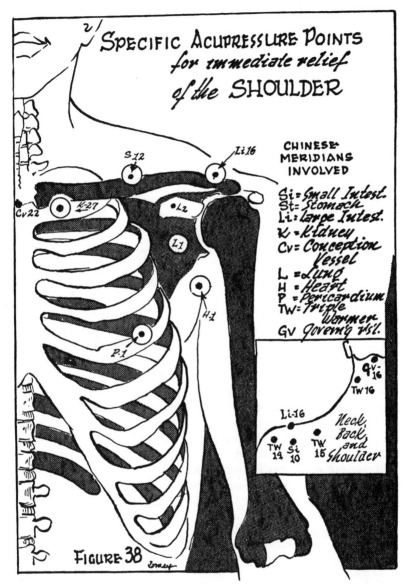

SPECIFIC ACUPRESSURE POINTS
for immediate relief
of the SHOULDER

CHINESE
MERIDIANS
INVOLVED

Si = *Small Intest.*
St = *Stomach*
Li = *large Intest.*
K = *Kidney*
Cv = *Conception*
Vessel
L = *Lung*
H = *Heart*
P = *Pericardium*
TW = *Triple*
Warmer
Gv *Governing rsl.*

Neck,
Back
and
Shoulder

FIGURE 38

alongside those spinal bones and you will dispel the toxic waste that has collected there. Do this standing or sitting. In standing or sitting, at all times, do it without slouching or slumping.

In using acupuncture points up the spine to the neck, it becomes almost impossible to self-apply pressure. To use this million dollar health technique, there are two recourses. Either you have a buddy do it for you, or, lie on a golf ball. Simply lie back on the ball

Get yourself in such position that it comes right at the desired point. Lie back for the ten count and then inch up or down according to where you are starting. The ball remains stationary as possible. It's you who moves. The ball becomes a fulcrum or pressure contact. With your fingertips, now locate the tension areas between shoulders and neck. Note the knots. Press each. If you have a friend to do this for you, have him standing behind you (as you sit on a stool), placing his palms down on the scapular area, and apply pressure downwardly.

The SHOULDERS . . . Erasers of Fatigue

Technique for Figure 38

Fatigue collects in the shoulders as it does in other body parts. Muscles and joints and bursa sacs are the first to protest. Such fatigue-waste collections may be the result of systemic diseases, metabolic changes, glandular diseases, or even anemia. Bad posture, over-use, and accidents play a role.

When shoulder stiffness limits the use of the arm, you will find nodules of tension in the muscles of the shoulder, over the scapula, and on the upper arm. Apply *Acupressure, U.S.A.* Feel the muscle bodies wriggle beneath your fingertips as they disappear. Now shrug your shoulders as the muscles begin to loosen. Bring shoulders up to your ears. Now super-extend your head and bring your shoulders down. Direct your chin to the right shoulder. Then to the left.

Massage the muscles on the side opposite to the side to which the head is turned. This stretches the muscles. Now move to the upper chest muscles. Massage all areas in spasm. These are protest or fatigue areas. Eliminate them before they convert to "sprain" or "strain" during activity. These same "ouch spots" on the anterior of the chest wall may be harbingers of a future "heart attack." Check the front of the shoulder. Palpate for areas of pain. Use *Acupressure, U.S.A.* to advantage before descending the arm to the hands.

The HAND . . . Erasers of Fatigue

Technique for Figure 39

Weakness in the hands and arms too often indicates fatigue rather than nerve involvement or muscular deficiency. It indicates collections of toxic waste piling up in the soft tissues, and *Acupressure, U.S.A.* is the technique of choice to release it. Starting

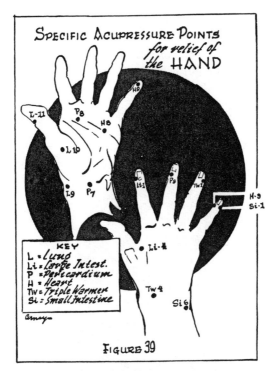

SPECIFIC ACUPRESSURE POINTS *for relief of the* HAND

KEY
L = *Lung*
Li = *Large Intest.*
P = *Pericardium*
H = *Heart*
Tw = *Triple Warmer*
Si = *Small Intestine*

FIGURE 39

at the fingertips, grasp the fingertip and pull. Then use a rotary motion of the thumb on the top of each finger joint. (With the index finger underneath, and the thumb on top, this treats both sides of the fingertip at the same time.) *Acupressure, U.S.A.* effectively treats dormant glands by way of the meridians that are in each finger. For example, the *Small Intestine meridian* begins just behind the fingernail of the little finger.

The *Triple Warmer meridian* begins just behind the nail on the dorsum of the fourth finger. The *Large Intestine meridian* has its inception at the dorsum and tip of the index finger. On the palmar side, the *Lung meridian* is in the thumb, the *Pericardium* or *"Circulation-Sex" meridian* is in the third finger, and the *Heart meridian* is in the fifth finger. Each goes to the fingertips. With this in mind, pressure on the fifth little finger helps people with "heart trouble."

People with weak little fingers usually have a heart problem of one kind or another, according to the Orientals. People with strong thumbs, they also indicate, are very often "brainy" people, as well as manually strong. Treatment, via *Acupressure, U.S.A.* on the third finger, is beneficial to people with high blood pressure. This procedure stimulates the sex organs and is good also for those with a problem of the intestines.

There is one very important acupuncture point on the palm of the hand and another in the web between index finger and thumb.

Look at the palm of your hand. Note the heart line. Now look

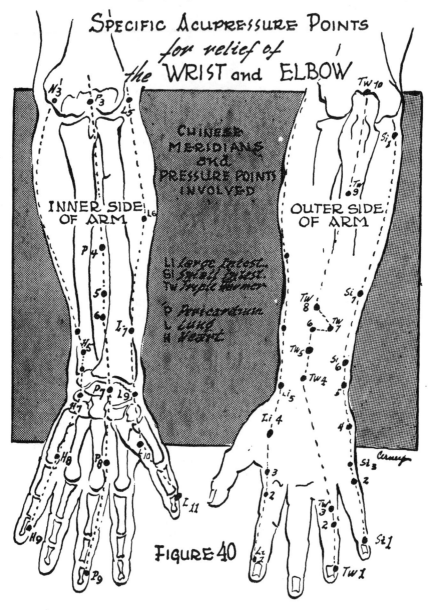

FIGURE 40

at the point where the fourth and fifth fingers join. It is behind the web, immediately over the heart line, that you make contact for rotary motion and pressure for all cardiac difficulties.

NOTE ... on CARDIAC (HEART) EMERGENCIES: *Where there has been cardiac arrest, or other emergency heart problem, grasp the tip of the little finger* (both hands) *and simply whirl it around. This emergency health care has been known to save more than one life, and by using the Oriental approach to the Heart meridian, you utilize and inspire the very lifeline to living.*

Now return to acupuncture point H-8. Place your thumb on the palm at this point and your index finger immediately opposite on the back of the hand. Note the tenderness. Massage as you compress and you will not only help the heart but energize yourself as well!

The WRIST and ELBOW . . . . . Erasers of Fatigue

Technique for Figure 40

Grasp the wrist between thumb and index finger. Locate tenderness areas in the wrist. Apply acupressure wherever you locate pain. Move up the arm in steps (1½ inches apart) on the outside of the arm toward the elbow. Just below the elbow is another *sanri*. Whether this point is tender or not, stimulate this energizer before continuing your excursion toward the shoulder. Repeat the process on the other arm.

Use these acupuncture points and meridians to your advantage in disposing of fatigue in your body. Learn the message they have to tell. If the Li-4 acupuncture point is tender (where the thumb joins the index finger), it indicates that your bowel is ailing. To get the larger intestine to improve, massage this point deeply. Then check along the thenar process (fat pad on the thumb side). If it is sensitive, it indicates the lungs are not functioning properly. Massage deeply and also get respiratory and digestion system benefits for releasing the toxic products of fatigue.

The ABDOMEN . . . . . Erasers of Fatigue

Technique for Figure 41

More ailments than we care to admit find their origin in the abdomen. If you would insure yourself of having a good day—free of fatigue—each day of your life, use your Pre-Breakfast seek-and-find

The ABDOMEN
and CHEST Schematically

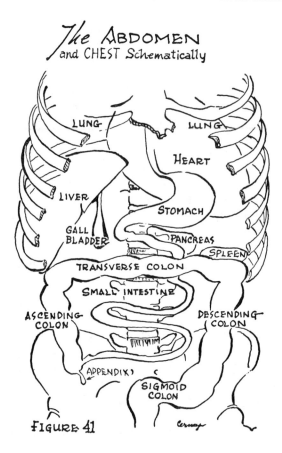

LUNG

LUNG

HEART

LIVER

STOMACH

GALL
BLADDER

PANCREAS

SPLEEN

TRANSVERSE COLON

SMALL INTESTINE

ASCENDING
COLON

DESCENDING
COLON

APPENDIX?

SIGMOID
COLON

FIGURE 41

routine indicated in Part I. This will not only help you determine which organ is laggard, but also which one to treat to get rid of toxic waste and fatigue. Use your Pre-Breakfast routine daily! Utilize those few moments lying in bed using *Acupressure, U.S.A.* as insurance against developing that stomach ulcer. Use it to improve your metabolism and to get your bowels to move on a regulated basis. Use it to assure yourself of improved health and more pleasant living.

In bed, on the floor, standing or sitting, use the following quickie techniques that can assure you of a wonderful day and get rid of the toxic elements that bring on fatigue.

QUICKIE TECHNIQUES
FOR REVITALIZATION

Solar Plexus Stimulus

Technique for Figure 42

To a slow three count, place the fingertips of both hands right into the solar plexus area. Hold. Release. This is acupuncture point 14 on the *Conception Vessel meridian* and point 22 of the *Kidney meridian*. This may not sound like much, but when you are dealing with the fantastic powers of regeneration and revitalization, you are dealing with power switches.

Now go to a point midway between the tip of your sternum and your belly button. Press! Hurt? Descend to a point midway between

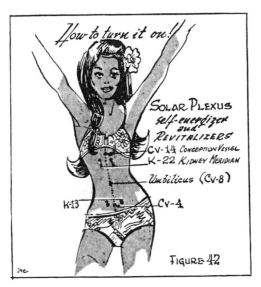

the umbilicus and your symphysis pubes. Press each of these areas for the three count. No more, no less. At this point, move slightly to the right on your lower abdomen. Hold for the three count. Move an inch over. Press. Then move another inch. Press. Do the same to the left. What you have done now is to innervate the *Kidney meridian* once again, as well as touch those magic keys to the *Stomach* and *Spleen meridians.*

Liver Stimulus

Technique for Figure 43

Curl the fingertips of both hands up under the right rib cage, right into the liver. Gently! At first it will hurt. As the condition of the liver improves, this hurt will go away and *this is your criterion of improvement*. Now move medially toward the body midline. At the point where the right ribs make an upward turn toward the breast bone, bury your finger once more in the abdomen. Hold for a three count and release. This innervates the gall bladder. It also helps chase the gas out of the hepatic flexure of the large colon, as well as activating the gall bladder.

Go across to the opposite side of the abdomen. Bury your fingertips in the area below the left ribs. Hold. Release. Maintain your three count slowly on each point of pressure. Remember that everything within the abdomen is controlled by nerve supply from

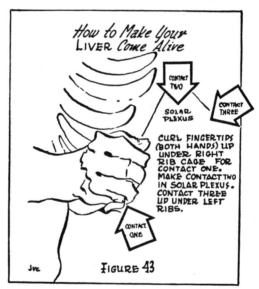

How to Make Your LIVER Come Alive

CONTACT TWO

SOLAR PLEXUS

CONTACT THREE

CURL FINGERTIPS (BOTH HANDS) UP UNDER RIGHT RIB CAGE FOR CONTACT ONE. MAKE CONTACT TWO IN SOLAR PLEXUS. CONTACT THREE UP UNDER LEFT RIBS.

CONTACT ONE

FIGURE 43

the spine. This means the spinal control buttons must also be pressed. For example, when there is a gall bladder involvement, there will be a painful spot between the shoulder blades. This is a reflex point, and it has to be eliminated. *Acupressure, U.S.A.* is your answer. How do you do it? Use that golf ball trick and lie back on it. Or, have a friend press his thumbs into it while you are lying face down. The areas of hurt will be between the fifth and ninth thoracic vertebrae.

NOTE: *Be gentle in your acupressure at all times. If there is pain at any one point, press gently until the hurt disappears. If pain remains unremittent, back off. Return another day.*

One more quickie move. How to relieve that cesspool of the abdomen called the "bowel"? Too often fatigue and disease begin right there! The entire length of the small and large intestines is a toxic retainer that has to be relieved of its contents. Here's the procedure to use.

Navel Stimulus

Technique for Figure 44

Place the tip of your third finger in your navel. Press deeply. Locate areas of pain. Now make circling excursions around the periphery of your umbilicus with slightly more pressure on the "ouch areas." Some of this pain may radiate in different directions.

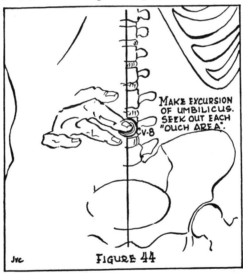

FIGURE 44

This radiation merely points to the exact place where a physical problem exists. These specific points will get more attention later.

This circular pressure technique around the navel will diminish the pain factor with each excursion and lower your fatigue level. Now place your hands palms down on your abdomen. Right hand on the right side, left on the left side. With your fingertips buried in the lower belly, pull up and push in toward the spinal column. Make ten rhythmic motions. With the fingertips still buried in the tissues, pull your lower belly up toward the rib cage. Be gentle but firm. You may feel and hear gurgling. Good. Lie there and relax. Then get up and drink hot water. Shortly thereafter, you will have a desire to go to the toilet. Repeat this routine each morning of your life, and you will live longer and stay younger day after day.

The CHEST . . . . . Erasers of Fatigue

Your next move is a seek-and-find mission. Run your fingertips across your chest wall above the breasts. Check for little "bumps," especially over the left breast (*not* in the breast). Massage these bumps out gently. These "bumps" are usually venous valves that are not working. Wherever such nodules exist, the person more often than not has, is about to have, or has had, heart trouble.

Move over toward the shoulder below the clavicle an inch or so. Probe. Does your thumb bring out a yip of pain? This is where the *Lung meridian* begins. This "alarm point" signals immediately when an ailment is going on in the lung. (See Figure 32.) If the hurt is on one side of the chest, you will also find it on the other side of your chest. Treat both sides. To do this, place your thumbs directly into the acupuncture point. Bring the elbows up and out. Make circles with your elbows. This rotary motion, silly as it may look, benefits the lungs. It is an important stimulus to respiratory action and the removal of fatigue and toxic waste.

The NECK . . . . . Erasers of Fatigue

Technique for Figure 45

The neck (side, front, and back) is vital not only to alleviating physical distress, but also is necessary to the elimination of fatigue each day of your life. The front and sides of your neck have three meridians coursing through, just under the skin: the *Stomach meridians* (two of them), running parallel upward on each side of the Adam's apple; the *Large Intestine meridian*, coursing upwardly and laterally to the stomach meridian; and from the chin downwardly (dead center), the *Conception Vessel meridian*. Posteriorly, on the back of the neck, are the *Bladder, Gall Bladder, Governing Vessel,* and *Triple Warmer meridians.*

Each one of them is in intimate control of organs and parts that can be stimulated and regulated to relieve fatigue. Sure, it looks complicated, but not with this book in your hand. Look at it this way: each one of these meridians is a lifeline to living; each is a

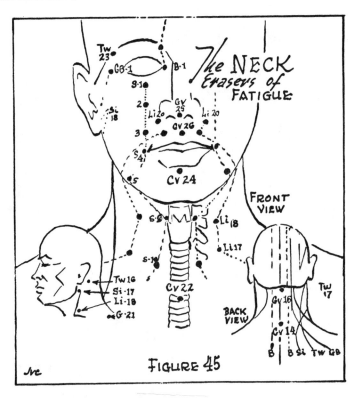

freeway to health—so use them to your advantage in relieving fatigue.

For example, if you are having trouble sleeping, and resultant fatigue-products have built up, you've got to do something about it, don't you? Well the neck, with a few other key areas, is the place to start. Here's how.

Technique for Figure 46

Point your index, third, and fourth fingers toward your Adam's apple. Use both hands. Press gently. Locate an area that throbs. This is your carotid artery. There's one on each side of the neck. If you don't feel it, you are in the wrong place. Move farther toward the center line. Good. Press. Hold for a slow three count. Release. Repeat three times. Now, with your thumbs, make stroking motions, from the jaw, down over the carotid artery.[1] Do it lightly, firmly, and *do not pause or press!*

Repeat three times first on the right side and then on the left.

---

[1] This procedure is also good for high blood pressure.

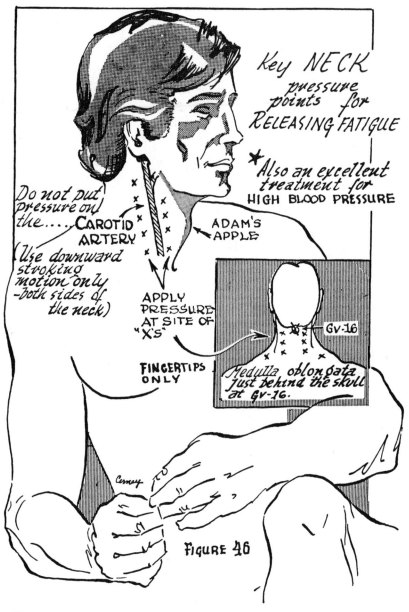

Key NECK pressure points for RELEASING FATIGUE

* Also an excellent treatment for HIGH BLOOD PRESSURE

Do not put pressure on the.... CAROTID ARTERY (Use downward stroking motion only —both sides of the neck)

ADAM'S APPLE

APPLY PRESSURE AT SITE OF "X's"

FINGERTIPS ONLY

Gv-16

Medulla oblongata just behind the skull at Gv-16.

FIGURE 46

Now go to the back of the neck. At the base of the skull, midline on the neck, is a hollow. In front of that hollow—inside the skull—is an all-important part of the nervous system called the *medulla oblon-*

gata. Note the tenderness in this hollow as you insert the third finger of each hand. Press for the three count. Pause. Repeat three times. Now move an inch to either side. You will note additional tenderness zones or "ouch spots." Muscles attach in the skull at this point. Apply pressure in the same manner. Now go to the *Bladder meridian* as indicated in Figure 45. It runs just under the skin over the trapezius muscle.

Two More Steps

Technique # 1

With the thumb and index finger, probe the web between the thumb and index finger on your other hand. Sensitive? Is there a knot or bump? Use a thumb and index finger rotary pressure on it until it dissolves. This special point not only relieves the *Large Intestine meridian* of toxic waste but it is vital in treating insomnia. Use it on yourself each night and note the benefits as fatigue simply melts away. Note how much better you sleep!

Technique # 2

In your desire to sleep better to get rid of fatigue, return now to your neck. Stroke the carotid arteries, as indicated earlier, three times. Breathe deeply. Press your fingertips into that hollow at the base of the skull once more. Now stretch your arms and legs. Stretch! STRETCH! Relax. Blank your mind of everything. Sleep. Let Nature take its course, and by way of *Acupressure, U.S.A.* and the "magic buttons" of the Oriental meridians, will fatigue melt away.

HOW TO GET RID OF
THAT TIRED FEELING

3

Fatigue is usually a state of mind rather than of body. Not always. Boredom as well as overwork may bring it on. No matter how or where it develops, there *is* a method you can use to restore that feeling of well-being so vital to "feeling great." By using *Acupressure, U.S.A.* you can get rid of that tired feeling, and all it takes is *one minute!* One minute! Sixty seconds, to revitalize and step yourself up for action—and I'm going to show you how.

If a few hours at work make you tired, if morning finds you weary after a full night's sleep, if you are quickly bored by your job, then you need an *Acupressure, U.S.A.* "booster shot." You need the kind of self-treatment that helps you get rid of toxic waste in your system and sets the *ch'i* (energy) flowing in the meridians. Remember that fatigue does not mean too little sleep. It means your meridians—your energy channels—are stagnant. Therefore, it's up to you to start that energy going. It's up to you to start the dynamo as set out in this book.

How a Television Star
Got Her "Booster Shot"
and Lost That Tired Feeling

Maria M., playing a leading role in a television "soap opera," was one of those getting that "tired feeling." Her dynamos had run down. She, like all people in show business, and in all other industries, are subject to "let-downs." To cope with the problem, some people resort to alcohol, drugs, or other stimulants. Actress Maria M. was no exception. This lovely little woman was on a grueling shooting schedule. Although she had the weekends off, she was spending 14 to 18 hours a day in the studio and was simply wearing out. At 52 she couldn't cut the mustard like she did when she was an ingenue on Broadway. When I saw Maria she wasn't just tired. Her face was gaunt. Pancake makeup didn't hide the lines. She cried when she saw what camera closeups were doing. Her producer suggested rest but wouldn't give her leave of absence. She tried getting the writers to write her out of the script temporarily. This didn't work. They said she was the one who was "carrying" the show. Worn out, nervous, exploding over everything and anything, she came to my office. We worked out a plan of action. Here's the program I suggested.

One Minute Work-Out for Generating Self-Power

STEP 1: Rub your hands briskly (palms and fingers) (five seconds).

STEP 2: Now rub your warmed palms up and down on your cheeks. Do it briskly (five seconds). Then. . .

STEP 3: Pitter-pat the top of your head with the flat of your hands in a five-second tattoo. This provides a molecular bombardment of stimulation to the meridians under the scalp.

STEP 4: Cup the hand in a loosely bound fist. Tap vigorously up and down the inside and outside of each arm (three excursions are sufficient).

STEP 5: Gently apply pressure on the thyroid gland (below the Adam's apple area) between thumb and index finger. Three times only.

STEP 6: Press on one carotid artery for the count of five. Release. Breathe deeply. Re-apply. Go to the other side of the neck and repeat.

STEP 7: Place your thumb in the hollow at the base of your skull (at midline where head sits on spinal column). Press. Hold for three count. Release. Repeat three times. Then go to the feet.

STEP 8: Techniques for the feet:

    a. Pinch the tip of the great toe. Then compress the ball of the big toe. You will note a sharp, painful spot. Rub it away.

    b. Place your thumb in the kidney reflex zone (see Figure 22). Hold. Release. Re-apply.

    c. Grasp the Achilles tendon tightly. Hold. Release. Repeat three times on each extremity.

    d. Briskly rub the top of the foot with your hand. Or,

more conveniently, with the heel of the other foot.

STEP 9: With the palms open, slap the lower extremities—front, side, and back, from foot to groin.

PRECAUTION: *Do not use this step if varicose veins are present!*

As you go through this 60-second work-out, you will note a general warmth suffusing you, a feeling of well-being. You have stimulated the power stations. All systems are at Go. So go! It's the only one-minute "break" in the world that's worth a million!

HOW TO GET RID
OF TENSION

What does tension have to do with acupuncture with or without needles? Everything! Acupuncture points become sensitive when there is feed-back through the autonomic nervous system. The brain is a part of this system. Aggravations, frustrations, insecurity, fear, all play a role—along with organic ailments—in sensitizing that alarm center called an acupuncture point.

Just as heart trouble may begin with stress and tension, so do headaches, morning fatigue, and high blood pressure. All have their inception in emotions and "nerves." The greater the emotional conflict, the greater the tension. The more the tension, the more this neuro-genic force will be apt to collect in—and begin to destroy—the integrity of some central organ. As the organ begins to ail, it shunts its message of hurt out to the skin, where lie the acupuncture points. These points become tender to touch.

The power and speed of these forces is amazing. For instance, previously healthy businessman John D. watched in agony as his life's savings and his business went down the drain due to a partner absconding with the funds. He got stomach ulcers. His skin aged. His hair turned grey. His eyes lacked luster. His mind dulled. He became an old man almost overnight. In a matter of six months tension laid him low, and he could have licked this vicious cycle with *Acupressure, U.S.A.*

Then there was actor Hale N. It was the sundown years of his career. The studios wanted only the younger generation, and this put knots in his belly. Then came diarrhea followed by constipation, and all of it was a sign of how tensions had converted to an organic expression called *colitis*. It was all tension. Tension leaves its mark. If you look for these semaphore signals, you can stop them from going further by treating yourself with *Acupressure, U.S.A.* and bringing yourself back to health!

If you don't believe you have tensions, examine yourself the next time you stop for a red light and the car behind you starts blowing its horn even before the light has changed! Did you note the sudden knot in your gut? See your fists clench? Teeth grind? Of course you have! It's a normal reaction of anger and fight. It's the body's response to emotion. It's tension!

Quickie Technique
for Emergency Handling
of Tension

Reach back to the base of your skull. Place the third finger of each hand into the hollow at the base of your skull. Rotate them around. Note the pain. Now move to the right of this hollow. Note the bump. It too will be tender. It may be downright painful on pressure. Give it *Acupressure, U.S.A.* Repeat on the other side of the hollow. Now, with your head bowed forward, run each hand firmly down the back of your neck toward the shoulders. Repeat five times. By diplomatic persuasion of the acupuncture points and Chinese meridians, you will have released your tensions in a matter of seconds.

How Is Acupressure, U.S.A.
an Answer to Tension?

Our Oriental friends have already proven that pain can be controlled. This also applies to tensions. Pressure on given points on the neck can bring beneficial reactions with no trail of drug disaster, no trail of hurt from unnecessary surgery—but rather miracles of healing that make human beings whole again!

How to Run a Tension-Test
On Yourself

If you have an element of doubt about the use of acupuncture or acupressure centers, and how all these superficial points are connected with internal organs, whether they be brain, chest, or abdominal, let's make an experiment. You have a surprise coming!

Test One

Insert your right index finger into the hollow behind your right ear lobe. Get it in there! Rotate! Hurt? Under normal circumstances, there is no hurt. In tense people, this is a point of pain. It is an acupuncture point awaiting therapy. Try the other side of your neck. Less painful? More painful than the other side? Surprise you? But these are the intimate details you will be getting in this book. Some of what you learn will surprise you. In fact, in the learning, you will relieve your own headaches, your own sinus problems, and create unanticipated little miracles of your own.

Test Two

In seated position, lay your head toward one shoulder. On the exposed side, run your fingers firmly down the heavy muscle extending from the base of the skull to the shoulder. Note little bumps in the muscle enroute. Locate each. Note their hard, rounded texture. Each is a knot of tension. Each is a point of fatigue. Repeat on the opposite side of the neck.

Now that you have located the tension areas, acupress each until the little knots of tension disappear under your fingertips. Now move up the muscle to the base of the skull to its insertion. You will find a somewhat swollen, soft bump. These too are key spots. Sink your third finger into each, one by one. Sit back. Relax. Note the blissful feeling of relaxation that pervades you. Accomplish this and you are on your way, not just to conquering *Acupressure, U.S.A.*, but to restoring yourself to a new degree of health. You are using *acupuncture without needles* in a method that I call "Acupressure" and the Chinese call *T'ui-na, an-mo,* and *chien-an.*

In testing these trigger points, mark them first with a skin pencil or ballpoint pen. "X" marks the spot until you are totally familiar with how they feel and where they are. Treat with rotating fingertip pressure up to one minute. Unless scar tissue is present, many of these areas of distress will dissolve beneath your fingertips. Tension knots of long standing will want to refuse to depart. This is often noted in "whiplash" injuries.

SUSTAINED GO-POWER
AND HOW TO GET IT WITH ACUPRESSURE, U.S.A.

Everyone needs go-power today. Everyone needs stamina.

Everyone is looking for the magic elixir that will give them sustained drive, and they need look no further than the hidden dynamos that are within them. Within you is the most fabulous machine in the world for creating and maintaining high-power energy. It's a God-given power, and all you have to do is utilize it. All you have to do is press the buttons that turn on a dynamo of action.

In this particular instance, you begin with that little hollow between two muscle attachments at the base of your skull. Put your finger into that central area. Feel it! Probe it! Painful? Exactly! What is this fantastic button? What is it capable of doing to give you sustained go-power so that you can swim the deepest ocean, climb the highest mountain, run faster than anyone else in the world?

Medulla Oblongata: Your Power Station

Technique for Figure 47

In that magic hollow at the base of the skull is a vitality-generating acupuncture point. It's called Gv-16 on the Oriental charts, or, the 16th acupuncture point in the *Governing Vessel meridian*. It lies just on the other side of the skull from the dynamo within. That dynamo is called the *medulla oblongata*.

The medulla oblongata is that enlarged portion of the spinal cord just after it enters the cranium. As a giant controlling agent, it contains the respiratory center and the cardiovascular center. It integrates the reflexes concerned with swallowing and vomiting. It controls postural balance. It controls blood pressure and the dilation and constriction of blood vessels. It has many more duties, but the factor of importance here is that any therapy applied to this area—even though on the outside of the skull—is going to cause reactions.

Pressure at Gv-16 not only relieves tensions but steps up vitality. It "turns on the juice" for making the body more capable of sustained action. The entire human nerve network is funneling impulses into it. These messages are relayed to the power-manufacturing centers of the brain and body. The message goes to the thyroid gland and the pituitary, to the adrenal glands that reside on the kidneys. Each of these glands is a source of giant power; each one is a producer of giant-making hormones; each in its own way is a manufacturer of stamina, with the power to regulate every body cell and maintain it for a lifetime.

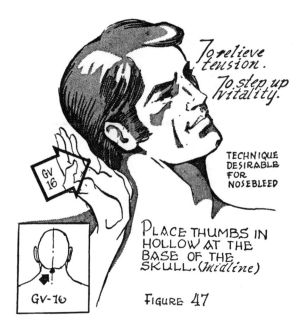

To relieve tension.
To step up vitality.

TECHNIQUE DESIRABLE FOR NOSEBLEED

GV 16

PLACE THUMBS IN HOLLOW AT THE BASE OF THE SKULL. (Midline)

GV-16

FIGURE 47

When you apply *Acupressure, U.S.A.* into that hollow at the base of the skull, you are on a direct line with those powerhouses via the medulla oblongata.

If you would develop stamina, utilize Gv-16 at the base of your skull. If you are going to climb that highest mountain, make that biggest sale, compete in a 100-yard dash; if you are an actor going on for your big performance; if you are a housewife who needs a lot of go-power to keep ahead of things at home—use your head! Use your medulla oblongata which affects all these powerhouses and makes energy available on command!

How to Call up Secondary Shock
Troops for Courage and Fight-Power

At your very fingertips are control buttons, pressure points, on the neck and upper back, that can be used to give you that little bit extra, that "booster shot" so vital to winning. Those acupuncture points are on either side of the cervical (neck) vertebrae and those vertebrae of the back (lumbars and thoracics). To utilize *Acupres-*

sure, U.S.A. properly for this purpose, locate first on the neck a muscle that extends forwardly and down from the mastoid process back of your ear, attaching at the breastbone. This muscle is called the *sternocleidomastoid* muscle. We'll use this as the guideline for your thumb and other fingers, which, when compressed, will be making contact on four important meridians (*Stomach, Large Intestine, Small Intestine,* and *Triple Warmer meridians*).

With your right hand, now make contact with your thumb at the base of your throat. Plant your other fingers on the back of the neck. Squeeze. Move up an inch. Squeeze. Move up inch by inch until you get to the skull. Then do the left side. To save time, both may be done at the same time with opposite hands. Make two total excursions; it takes less than ten seconds to do it.

Now find a doorframe. Get your right upper back—between the shoulder blade and spinal column—up against the protruding edge of the frame. Move your feet forward so that you are creating pressure backwardly. This pressure will unearth some "ouch spots." Expect them. In position, move from side to side as if scratching your back. Then repeat on the opposite side of the spinal column.

In doing this, note the warm flush in your face. This immediate vasomotor reaction is taking place all over your body inside and out. You are being flooded with power values. You are being energized, and all you are doing is taking advantage of standard equipment Nature has made available to you at all times.

HOW TO HANDLE
AILMENTS IN THE HEAD

4

HEADACHES
AND HOW TO HANDLE THEM

Pain in the head is a symptom common to many illnesses. Handling a headache properly depends on its cause in terms of regular westernized medicine, but in *Acupressure, U.S.A.* the approach is entirely different.

How Mary Lee Conquered Her Headaches

Mary Lee S. had been under psychiatric care for her headaches before she came to me. She'd been to clinics and top specialists in the field. In her 30's, her headaches were so terribly painful her personality changed. She lost her friends. She lost her husband, and then lost her job because of it. In doing an in-depth history and examination, I found her remarkably free of physical problems, yet, day after day, there it was—headache, ranging from mild to severe, off-again, on-again pain.

Her previous physicians all had different diagnoses. One diagnosed her headaches as being due to an ovarian cyst. One said a gall bladder operation was immediately necessary. One said she was allergic to dust and pollen. Another said that what she needed was an environmental change. In my own case, I simply couldn't tie down a cause until I checked the meridians on her abdomen. They were wildly positive, and yet all other tests were negative. Acupuncture therapy was begun, and in one week the headaches were gone. Her bowels were moving regularly. She was sleeping at night. Her energy level came back, and for her it was a little miracle. Today Mary Lee is happy and well. Her normally sweet personality has returned. She's back on her old job and her husband has returned home. At home now, she uses *Acupressure, U.S.A.* and maintains that beautiful state of well-being called health.

HEAD PAIN ... AND
HOW TO UNDERSTAND IT

For a better awareness of why taking an aspirin for a headache is not always the best thing to do, let's look at some of the more complex aspects of head pain. Let's point out that some head pains may come from outside the skull as well as from within. Head pains may be due to such a thing as a brain abscess or an infection of the meninges.

It may be due to hemorrhage or tumor. Headaches may be due to changes in the very bones of the skull itself. It may be due to something wrong with the sensory nerves in the scalp or to circulatory disturbances, such as in high blood pressure, infections, or allergies. It may be due to a blow on the head or the back of the neck. Head pain may be due to hysteria, anxiety, or other mental stress.

What I'm getting at is that getting rid of pain in the head is one thing, but if you are taking aspirin or other drugs for the headache when actually more yeoman care is necessary, then you'd better let your doctor determine the cause. He knows more about the matter than do you.

Headaches Have Many Causes

Headaches *do* have many causes and their location often identifies their course. Like many other physical pains, this is not always true. Headaches are never confined to any one nerve or part unless it's migraine. For your convenience and understanding, a list of head pains is catalogued in Figure 48.

The Character of Head Pain

Head pain varies with people and with cause. With Mary Lee S., it was a stabbing, drilling, or lancing pain. With John D., it was sharp and confined as in neuralgia. With Francis K., her head pain pulsated and throbbed on one side and sometimes invaded both sides. Bartender Mac S.'s headache was dull, diffused, and "heavy" as a result of general infection. Jeannie J.'s headache was of the squeezing or pressure type that occurs in neurasthenia and neurotic people. It was like a constricting band around her skull. Then there's the hot,

OCCIPITAL PAIN

(1) DYSPEPSIA
ADENOIDS
MIDDLE EAR AILMENT
BAD TEETH
EYE STRAIN
EMOTIONAL TENSION
PELVIC ORGAN DISEASE
NEURASTHENIA
SPINAL DISEASE
EPILEPSY
CEREBELLAR TUMOR
CERVICO- OCCIPITAL
          MYALGIA

EYEBALLS

(4) NEURALGIA (5ᵗʰ Nerve)
CORYZA (runny nose)
MIGRAINE HEADACHE
OPHTHALMOPLEGIA
INFLAMMATION - IRIS,
    CORNEA, CONJUNCTIVA

TOP OF HEAD

(5) HYSTERIA
ANEMIA
DISEASES OF OVARIES,
    BLADDER, UTERUS
NEURASTHENIA

UPPER JAW

(6) DENTAL PROBLEMS
ANTRUM DISEASES
CANCER
PERIOSTITIS
NEURALGIA (Superior
    Maxillary nerve)

LOWER JAW

(7) TEETH
MUMPS
NEURALGIA (Inferior
    Maxillary Nerve)

SIDE OF HEAD

(2) TEETH
OTITIS MEDIA (EAR)
FOREIGN BODY IN EAR
EYE STRAIN
CANCER OF TONGUE
ANEURYSM (INNOMINATE)
DISEASED MAXILLARY
    or TEMPORAL BONES

FRONTAL -
TEMPORAL

(3)
ANEMIA | DYSPEPSIA
EYES | CONSTIPATION
TEETH | UREMIA
DISEASED FRONTAL
          SINUSES
NEURASTHENIA
NEPHRITIS

HEAD PAIN and
ITS SOURCES

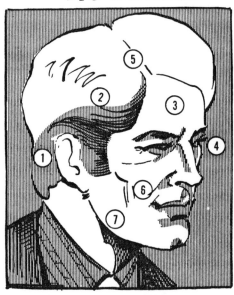

*Diagnostic indications,
your doctor looks for when
you have a headache.*

FIGURE 48

burning headache and sore scalp that fashion designer Klaus had as the result of his rheumatism and anemia.

Then there was Josephine J. who had sharp needle-like pains in her head and a burning sensation due to hysteria—and all of them, because they were educated to "take something to get rid of it"—were living on aspirin or other drugs, when *Acupressure, U.S.A.* would have been of greater help.

The Point Is,
Should We Constantly
Mask Pain with Pills?

"Because headaches have many causes," says Dr. Paul Word-man, "never forget that an aspirin tablet may be exactly what you *don't need* in controlling pain. Aspirin merely masks discomfort. It does nothing for its cause. Because of this, you must leave the diagnosis (where pain is unremitting) to your physician. Advise him as to the location of the pain, its character and intensity. After examination, let *him* determine what should be done!"

Location of Pain Is Important

Head pain may be temporal, frontal, parietal, occipital, or may even be in a vertical band around the skull, as indicated earlier. The headache of anemia is usually in front of the head as in constipation, but it may be on top even while the back of the head feels like it has just been rammed in—and all this makes for confusion.

Other Causes of Head Pain

In the headaches of nephritis (inflamed kidneys), pain may be due to poison in the bloodstream such as in uremia or other infections in the renal system. It may be due to that process of aging called "arteriosclerosis," in which blood vessels harden making it difficult to get blood supply to the brain. There may be tinnitus (ringing or other sounds in the head). The pain may throb. People with throbbing in their ears sometimes express vague fears and forebodings. Martin Luther, the churchman, had Meniere's disease—a disease of the inner ear—and the sounds he heard in his head shaped the vehemence of his preachments.

Jean's headache was usually worse in the morning as the result of her neurasthenia and tended to disappear in the afternoon. Headaches may come from swollen or infected turbinates of the nose and sinuses of the face. Such a head pain may start at the root of the nose and go backwardly to the rear of the head. Coughing, stooping, or bending, makes it worse.

Eyes may be a source of pain that hits the front of the head or the back. Headaches may come from indigestion and/or constipation. Such headaches are of the pulsating or throbbing type and are worse in the frontal and orbital areas. Sudden movement of the head emphasizes this pain.

When thinking about how pains may refer to faraway parts, it's interesting to note that in diseases of the uterus there may be sharp, radiating pain in the back of the head as well as in the breast and thigh. Pain may also occur in the ankle, and this too is one of the pressure or acupuncture "points" on a Chinese meridian that connects these parts. What I am pointing out is that *local head pain may have its inception somewhere other than in the head*, and of this you must be sharply aware. It is for this reason that *treatment for headache is never primarily local*, so use your *A B C Schedule of Action* efficiently. Use only as directed to get the best results.

HEADACHE CONTROL
A B C SCHEDULE OF ACTION

A	B	C	D	E	F
GB-15	TW-16	L-8	Liv-3	St-36	Sp-1

(See Figures 49, 50 and 65)

Explanation of
Contact Points

(A) Locate acupuncture point approximately four finger widths above each eye brow.

(B) Squeeze bridge of nose.

(C) Locate "ouch area" in hollow behind and below each ear.

(D) Pressure over radial (wrist) artery.

(E) Outside of knee, approximately three finger widths below level of knee cap or just above, and medial to the proximal head of the fibula.

(F) Dorsum of each foot at articulation of first and second metatarsals.

(G) Medial and lateral sides of the big toes and underneath in the fleshy part. Locate the "ouch area." Massage it until the hurt is gone. Then move down the foot relieving all other "ouch spots" you find.

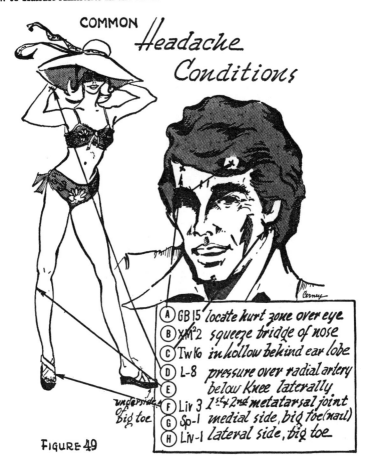

COMMON *Headache Conditions*

A) GB 15 *locate hurt zone over eye*
B) XM 2 *squeeze bridge of nose*
C) Tw 16 *in hollow behind ear lobe*
D) L-8 *pressure over radial artery below knee laterally*
E)
F) Liv 3 *1st + 2nd metatarsal joint* — *underside of big toe*
G) Sp-1 *medial side, big toe (nail)*
H) Liv-1 *lateral side, big toe*

FIGURE 49

Auxiliary
Techniques
for Headaches

(H) *Vortex-of-the-head pressure.* Note that Gv-21 at the top of the skull is particularly tender. Other zones will also be tender along the midline of the skull. With fingers in a row along this imaginary line, apply pressure. Repeat at least five times. Press. Hold. Release. You are now working on that all-important Chinese wonder-working meridian called the *Governing Vessel.*

(I) *Locate key painful point parallel to midline.* Find painful areas in your scalp with your fingertips. With four fingers on either side of the centerline on the skull—and parallel to this midline—

How to Use TRIGGER POINTS in treating HEAD PAIN

(TREAT BOTH SIDES OF HEAD IN) SAME MANNER

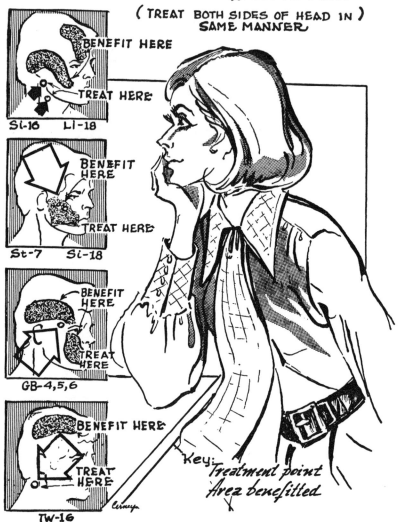

BENEFIT HERE

TREAT HERE

Si-16   Li-18

BENEFIT HERE

TREAT HERE

St-7   Si-18

BENEFIT HERE

TREAT HERE

GB-4,5,6

BENEFIT HERE

TREAT HERE

TW-16

Key:
Treatment point
Area benefitted

FIGURE 50

simply press your fingertips down and follow through by bringing the balance of your palm, or hand, down and press in at the temples. With this position, note that you have an actual grip on your scalp. Move it. Move it from back to front until it is loose. This will bring out residual pains in the centerline acupuncture points, so go back and compress them once more to release residual congestion and scalp contractions. You have been working with the *Bladder* and *Gall Bladder meridians.*

KEY ACUPUNCTURE POINTS
IN
"*TOU TONG*" HEADACHES BY ACCOMPANYING SYMPTOMS

Symptoms	A	B	C	D	E
When nose is clogged	Gv-16	B-12	Gv-23	Li-4	Tw-5
With vomiting, pain, and dizziness	GB-20	St-8	Gv-20	St-36 40	
Teeth as well as head hurts	GB-20	L-4	Liv-2		
Constant headache	B-17 18	St-36	T-23		
Intermittent pain at sides of head	GB-20	St-2 8	GB-14 41		Li-20

(See Figures 65, 95 and 96)

Supplementary Procedures

1. *Physical therapy application.*

   a. Massage muscles at back of neck and shoulders. Massage deeply into the abdomen and over the solar plexus.

   b. Stroke carotid arteries downwardly from below the jaw to the clavicles. Use your thumb on one side and other four fingers on the opposing side of the throat. Do it gently. This not only relieves brain congestion but stimulates the *carotid sinus.* This not only innervates the *Stomach meridian*, but the autonomic nervous system as well. Thus, via Americanized acupuncture, you relieve a nasty headache due to congestion, blood pressure malfunction, or even that headache due to emotions.

c. *Place icebag on top of skull* and a hot pack at the back of the neck.

d. *Avoid overexertion.*

e. *Keep the bowels cleaned out and the kidneys active.*

f. *Strong, black coffee* (very hot) where headache persists. *Do not use drugs of any kind!* Drink coffee *only* when headache is due to overstrain or fatigue.

g. *Get rid of the cause.* If headache persists, see your family doctor!

WHAT TO DO ABOUT MIGRAINE HEADACHES

Migraine headache is a periodic pain occurring usually on one side of the head, or along the course of the fifth cranial nerve. It may be accompanied by languor, chills, nausea, and disordered vision.

The true migraine headache has diversified origins, and seeking the cause is the name of the game. The Orientals feel that some migraines begin with the liver, with fear and tension; then when pain is in the temporal area, for example, it is due to the liver and gall bladder. When the pain shoots to the top of the head, it is due to the lack of proper function of the kidneys and bladder. When alcoholic hangovers play a role in migraine headaches, the treatment is more complex. In working out a schedule of treatment for migraine headaches, I developed a chart that simplifies the matter at a glance.

Maria D. had recurrent pains on one side of her head. Along with the head pain, she was depressed, irritable, and restless. Most of the time her headache remained localized. Sometimes it diffused all over the head. Along with it came vomiting, anorexia (loss of appetite), and tingling sensations. Her scalp was so tender she couldn't get her comb through her hair. Muscles in the back of her neck knotted up until she felt like her head was being drawn down into her shoulders.

Looking for relief, Maria toured the gamut of doctors, clinics, and hospitals. Her pain continued. Every time she menstruated, every time there was an emotional problem, whenever she was tired or had been using her eyes too much, there it was! Migraine . . . in full bloom! Certain foods brought it on. She might have an attack once or twice a year, or maybe two or three a week. In between the "attacks," there were no other symptoms. When I first saw her, she was frantic with pain. Emergency care was rendered immediately.

In the meantime, I wrote for and received reports from the hospitals in which she had been a patient. Obviously, her doctors had run complex tests and examined her for a cerebral accident, tumors, aneurysms, and even multiple sclerosis. They had run histamine tests and checked her accessory sinuses, made head x-rays, and did an encephalogram. All negative! In my own history-taking, I noted that Maria had no head pain the entire time she was pregnant. She also started having her "migraine" headaches about the time of puberty.

In other words, the whole problem seemed to hinge on endocrine influence. Her glands had to be playing a role in those awful headaches. The pituitary and ovaries *had* to be involved. With this key in mind, I began therapy. Her ABC SCHEDULE OF ACTION for migraine is as follows (see Figures 51 and 52):

**Here's How to Knock
the Head off Migraine**

A B C SCHEDULE OF ACTION

A	B	C	D	E	F	G	H
XH-3	GB-1,3	Tw-23	B-1	Li-4	L-6	Liv-2	Big Toe

(See Figure 52)

**Explanation of
Contact Points**

(A) Locate and gently compress the hollow area of the temples (XH-3). *Do not* compress the artery.

(B) Outer corner of each eye (GB-1, 3).

(C) In the hollow at ends of each eye brow (Tw-23).

(D) Compress medial corner of each eye (B-1).

(E) Dorsum of hand where thumb meets the index finger (Li-4).

(F) Outside L/R elbows (L-5).

(G) Lateral sides of great toe (Liv-2).

(H) Ball of big toe for pituitary gland reflex.

**Supplemental
Procedures**

1. *Institute prevention procedures.*
   a. Have eyes checked. Avoid excessive reading.

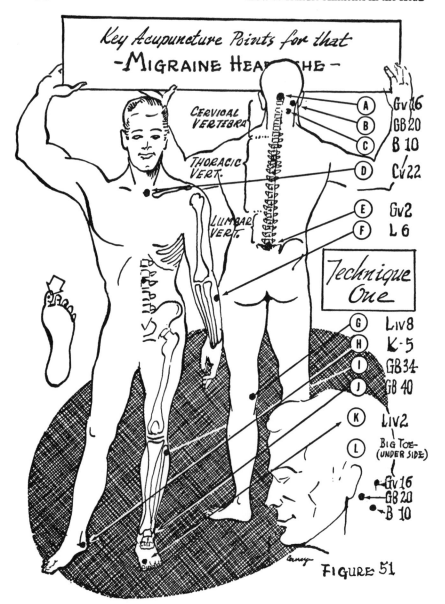

Key Acupuncture Points for that
— MIGRAINE HEADACHE —

Ⓐ	Gv 16
Ⓑ	GB 20
Ⓒ	B 10
Ⓓ	Cv 22
Ⓔ	Gv 2
Ⓕ	L 6
Ⓖ	Liv 8
Ⓗ	K-5
Ⓘ	GB 34
Ⓙ	GB 40
Ⓚ	Liv 2
Ⓛ	Big Toe (under side)

CERVICAL VERTEBRA

THORACIC VERT.

LUMBAR VERT.

Technique One

Gv 16
GB 20
B 10

FIGURE 51

b. Plenty of rest.

c. Purge weekly with saline solution (1 tablespoon salt per 1 quart of water).

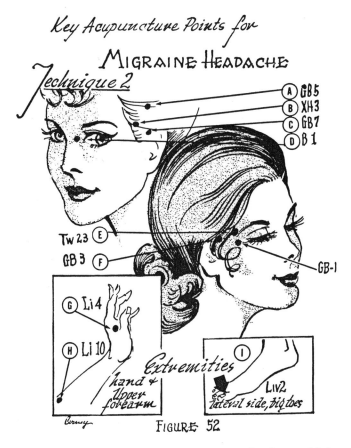

Key Acupuncture Points for

MIGRAINE HEADACHE

Technique 2

(A) GB5
(B) XH3
(C) GB7
(D) B 1

Tw 23 (E)
GB 3 (F)

GB-1

(G) Li 4
(H) Li 10

hand & upper forearm

Extremities

(I)

Liv2
lateral side, big toes

FIGURE 52

d. Eliminate from diet all known foods to which you are allergic.

e. Prior to the menstrual "period" (if female), rest with coldpack or icebag at the base of the skull.

f. Eliminate all drugs.

2. *During an "attack," rest in a darkened room. Be sure it is quiet, cool, well-ventilated.*

3. *Dietary supplementation:* add vitamin D and E to your diet.

4. *Avoid* overwork, alcohol, tea, coffee.

5. *Systematic exercise* daily (half hour).

6. *Bathe frequently.* Do *not* lay in hot tub! Utilize lukewarm shower, and end with a stimulating cold one. Rub down vigorously with a rough towel.

HEAD COLDS AND
THE "COMMON COLD"

The most common of all ailments is the "uncommon cold." Often referred to by physicians as "upper respiratory infection," it is an acute catarrhal involvement of one or more parts of the respiratory tract. In this particular case, we're concerned with the "head."

The exact cause for the "cold" has not yet been determined, yet the cause is transmitted with ease. It promptly affects those whose body resistance is down. Although its beginnings seem to be abrupt, it actually takes time to get incubated in people whose resistance is down. Once it takes hold, it may range from red nose to complete head and chest involvement.

Mamie D. came into my office with all the harbingers of the "common cold." She had headache and tickling and a scratchy feeling in her nose and throat, sneezing, and runny nose. She said, "I feel lousy." Her ability to smell and taste was impaired by the problem. She had transient aches in her back and extremities. A feeling of chilliness accompanied her fever. She had stood it as long as she could and then sought professional help. Along with office care I gave her instructions for home, and told her the big factor to remember in all acupressure and allied home therapy was that *symptoms* such as she had *may not be due to the common cold!*

Many illnesses such as diphtheria, meningitis, pharyngitis, whooping cough, and even measles *may be preceded by these same respiratory symptoms!* Hay fever, "grippe," influenza, allergies, may likewise set up the same train of symptoms. Where an actual head cold exists, here is the plan of action to cope with it.

How to Conquer
the "Common Cold"

A B C SCHEDULE OF ACTION

A	B	C	D	E
Tw-17	Gv-14 24	16 Li-20 4	Big Toe	9 St-10

(See Figure 53)

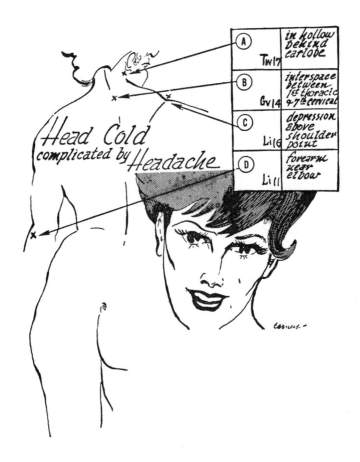

(A) Tw17	in hollow behind earlobe
(B) Gv14	interspace between 1st thoracic & 7th cervical
(C) Li16	depression above shoulder point
(D) Li11	forearm near elbow

Head Cold complicated by Headache

FIGURE 53

Explanation of Contact Points

(A) Locate hollow behind and below the ear (T-17).
(B) Midline at top of frontal bone (Gv-22).
(C) Either side of nose in the fold (Li-20).
(D) On the neck side of the shoulder point (Li-16).

Supplemental
Procedures

1. *Cold facts on "pressure point" ice therapy and how to treat
a "common cold."*

To supplement the strength of the acupuncture pressure
technique for various illnesses, I found ice singularly effective. For
the "common cold," I found that the application of ice prolonged
the capacity to control the "cold." My acupuncture technique was
aided immensely. For awhile, I thought the technique was unique to
the U.S.A. Then one day the *Washington Star* carried an article on
Dr. Menachem Ram of Rothschild Hospital in Haifa.

The story was about a "new invention" for curing the
"common cold." Dr. Ram's machine made low temperature applications and was described as being applied to the underside of the big
toes. Doctors Ram and his co-inventor, Aladar Schwartz of the Israeli
Institute of Technology in Haifa, admit *the treatment is akin to the
Chinese use of acupuncture.*

In the Oriental approach to human care, every body part is said
to have "an opposite number," which, when penetrated with a
needle, relieves the discomfort of its partner body part. In the case of
the "common cold," according to Dr. Schwartz, the nose and its
internal tissues, and the underside of the big toes, "appear to be
partners." Schwartz, an engineer, told newsmen he wasn't sure how
the "cold cure" worked, only that it did. He reported that of 100
cases treated, not one was a failure.

Having personally used the cold technique for the "common
cold" for over 30 years prior to their discovery, I can attest to the
value of their modern invention.

Cold Therapy Is Older
Than You Think

Low temperature, as an aid to acupuncture, and even as a
supplemental treatment for the "common cold," is *not new!* It's as
old as the mountains and the snow used to treat the wounds of
Alexander the Great, and the cold water that bathed the battle
wounds of the armed legions of Caesar's time in history.

Cold, as an anti-inflammatory agent and counter-irritant is also
a local analgesic. As an ancillary to *Acupressure, U.S.A.,* it provides

immediate surface cooling to relieve pain. It promptly soothes nose bleed or a burn. Coldpacks, wrapped around a sore throat, stop the swelling and diplomatically allay discomfort and pain. A coldpack lessens complications and after-effects in post-operative care. Most of all, it sets up autonomic system reactions that build the physical resistance necessary to conquer colds!

Realizing I could fortify acupuncture points with ice therapy, I have used it successfully over the years for such a problem as migraine headache for example, as well as for "colds." It works when drugs fail. It works when applied to acupuncture points. Along with helping the big problems, it is good for the treatment and relief of insect bites, lacerations, strains, sprains, and even poison ivy. Cold therapy, as old as time, is still a modern adjunct to the Americanized form of Chinese acupuncture called *Acupressure, U.S.A.* It's still my supplementary treatment of choice, and you too can use it as an aid to all physical therapy other than for the "common cold."

How to Make and Apply
Inexpensive Applicators

How may cold be best applied to acupuncture points? Simply freeze water in small, round-bottomed, plastic popsicle containers. Even more simply, *use an ice cube!* Apply the cube direct to the acupuncture pressure point with small circular motions. Gradually expand the circles until you are stroking more than the acupuncture area. Stroke gently for five minutes. Dry the part. Keep it warm. A favorable phenomenon will begin to take place.

Immediate Ice Massage . . .
Invaluable Aid to Acupuncture

Scientists have noted, as have I, that cold applications reduce muscle spasm, but no one has adequately described why the muscles relax or why a feeling of anesthesia exists after ice massage. *They simply haven't considered the acupuncture points and the meridians over which they are making icy contact!*

How to Get Rid of
the "Common Cold"

The next time you feel a "cold" coming on, conduct the following experiment! Take off your shoes and stockings. Probe the fat pad of your big toes. If the "cold" has not yet taken hold, these areas will demonstrate very little tenderness. As the infection begins to take over, the tenderness in your big toes gets worse. Now go to the top of your head. Note the sore spot right on the crown. Note that other spots in the scalp are also tender if other meridians, and the organs with which they are affiliated, have become involved. When these are extremely tender, the "cold" is full blown. But these are not only diagnostic points. Now go to work with Acupuncture, U.S.A. because these same acupuncture points will abort the problem you have!

Treatment That Brings
On Restful Sleep

Always fortify your acupuncture pressure point techniques with other procedures designed to help Mother Nature resist the invading foreign agents that cause any illness. Soak a turkish towel in cold water. Wring dry. Fold lengthwise in fourths and encircle the throat, if it is a "cold" or sore throat with which we are concerned. Replace as quickly as it warms. You will note a delightful warmth pervading your throat and body. Lassitude will steal over you. You will go to sleep. Remember that bed rest is one of the best combat agents for the common cold. Besides, it secludes you to prevent infecting others.

2. *Acupressure, U.S.A. therapy . . . and how-to-do-it techniques to knock out your cold.*

(a) *Finger pressure on neck (Stomach meridian 9-10).* Run your fingertips down both sides of your windpipe. Where one or more spots are specifically painful, pause, provide local pressure. If there is any hoarseness, this can be relieved, or prevented, by putting pressure on either side of the Adam's apple.

(b) *Thumb and index finger pressure on nose (XM-2).* Repeatedly compress and release nose from tip to bridge. As congestion breaks up, *do not blow your nose!* Drip dry. Wipe gently. (Blowing succeeds only in forcing bacterial agents back into the Eustachian tubes, which not only provides excellent bacterial-breeding headquarters but also infects the ear.)

(c) *Abdominal pressure points* for the "common cold." Apply fingers of both hands into the solar plexus (Cv-14) and liver area (G-24 and Sp-16). Press. Hold. Release. Breathe deeply and start again.

(d) *Spinal pressure release technique.* All persons with the "common cold" have a spinal problem in common. *All* of them will have tensions in the neck and shoulder muscles and demonstrate involvement of the thoracic vertebrae. No one in the world can demonstrate that this problem does not exist during the "common cold." So to help yourself to health, locate each one of these areas and use *Acupressure, U.S.A.!* How? Have a buddy apply his thumbs on each side of the vertebra that is expressing itself as an "ouch area." You lie face down. He applies his thumbs and leans forward on his arms to apply pressure. Or, if you are alone, apply the old golf ball trick. Simply lie back on the ball. Another technique I teach my patients is that of leaning back into a doorframe. Simply get the "ouch spot" on target and press.

As each of these methods goes into effect, you will feel results. If you are already in a bad way with a cold, don't expect miracles and immediate results. You will, however, have an accelerated recovery. If you feel a "cold" coming on, *prevent it!* Use *Acupressure, U.S.A.!* Use it regularly and you won't ever have a "cold," as acupressure specialists can attest by their own amazing experience in this field.

(e) *Dietary supplementation.* Take Vitamins A and D regularly. Take Vitamin C during the rainy and cold months. To date, all medical approaches to the "common cold" have been "shotgun therapy." Polybacterial vaccines are injected and the people still keep having colds. In fact, some react violently to the vaccine. The big problem in cold shots is this: *If you don't know what causes the problem in the first place, how can you treat it?* With vitamins, acupuncture, and acupressure, you are dealing with human resistance factors. You are dealing primarily with God's remedies. You are dealing with health!

3. *Drink copiously of water.*

4. *Bed rest if you can get away with it.*

YOUR FACE
AND HOW TO STAY LOOKING YOUNGER . . . LONGER

How a Prominent Business
Woman Stopped the Ravages
of "Change of Life"

Jan M. is a beautiful woman, and her mental brilliance is not the only thing unusual about her. In the business world, she's a genius. Advertising agencies are her field, and she's partner and executive vice-president of one of the best agencies in the U.S.A. She's a level-headed person, calm, adjusted, and has sustained go-power. She has something more—a million-dollar personality. She sells accounts that no one else can handle. When other account executives fail on a big deal, Jan is called in to take over. Her full breasts, lovely hips and legs, and peaches-and-cream complexion descend on a client like gangbusters, and within the hour she has his name on the dotted line. As simple as that. Jan was super girl!

Then something happened!

Super-girl fell apart! She didn't know what was happening at first and tried getting that "boost" via the cocktail route. Next it was "bennies." She was elbow deep in cigarette butts and coffee, and her usual lovely personality was gone. Like magic it disappeared, and more than her personality changed. Her breasts began to get flabby. Her belly potted. Unseemly hair began to show on her upper lip and the side of her face, and she simply "blew her cool." Her skin became lifeless, rough, scaly. Vitality was low. She was nervous, excitable, and had periods of terrible depression. Her muscles ached, her skin sweated and tingled. She simply couldn't sleep, and the pain in her low back and chest made her want to scream.

One of the hardest jobs I've ever had as a doctor was to tell this lovely lady that at the age of 28 she was going through premature change-of-life, that an infection she'd had a short time back had brought on a premature aging of the ovaries, that the traditional stage from 40 to 50 had already hit. Ovarian dynamos had gone to sleep and the ravages to youth were taking place.

Tears flowed. They were tears of desperation. First, because of her job. Secondly, because she was engaged to be married to a man whose one big dream it was to have children, and this was a crushing blow.

She Cried Out in Desperation

"What can I do?" she wanted to know. Her face was haggard. I recommended an excellent physician in the neighborhood who specialized in estrogenic therapy. I told her how it would help regulate the loss, but she thrust this suggestion aside. She reminded me that when she was doing research for a cosmetic account, she had estrogens used on her so that she could tell the women of the world her experience . . . through advertising . . . of exactly what it was like.

For Jan the results were unfortunate. She developed exquisitely sore breasts, vaginal bleeding, uterine cramps, abdominal bloating, and nervous tension that temporarily converted her into a shrew. From that point on, she was anti-medication of all kinds, and I guess that's why she became a patient of mine. Nature's ways are my only method of healing.

I suggested acupuncture and *Acupressure, U.S.A.* "Let's do it!" she exclaimed, and we did. Here was the program we followed.

SIX-POINT PROGRAM
FOR LOVELIER SKIN, EYE BEAUTIFICATION
BREAST BEAUTIFICATION, RELEASE OF
TENSIONS, AND IMPROVED HEALTH

**Oriental Techniques to
Achieve Your Desire for Beauty**

Skin Beautification

Technique for Figure 54. The magic ingredient *thyroxin* is released when you put pressure on the thyroid gland. This powerful endocrine substance travels freely in the bloodstream. This exotic power-hormone helps keep the skin soft, gentle in texture, and somewhat transparent. It revitalizes tissues so that the cheeks and neck do not sag and the lips remain full and firm.

For this purpose, acupress *Stomach meridian* acupuncture point 10 on either side of the lower neck. Remember that this is a very specific acupuncture point! It not only keeps the skin looking young, but *it keeps the hair from turning grey!*

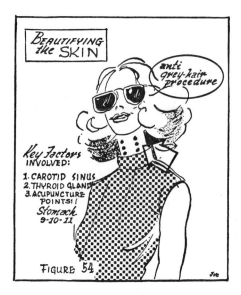

Eye Beautification

Technique for Figure 55. For that lovely, clear-eyed beauty, make index-fingertip pressure contact at the inside corner of each eye. This is *Bladder meridian* acupuncture point 1. Then go to the outside corner. This is *Gall Bladder meridian* 1. Both begin at the eye, and this makes them all-important points for stimulation. Now make a three-finger contact over the eye brows. (*Stomach* and *Bladder meridians* . . . St-1 and B-2.)

Now make forefingertip contact on TW-23 at the temples before going on to another magic area that marks a non-meridian point which traditional Chinese call *Nei Jing Ming*. Translation? "*Bright Eyes*," and these bright eyes can be yours by diplomatically and regularly applying *Acupressure, U.S.A.* on XH-4. Beauty . . . at your fingertips!

A Model's Case History

Joanie von D. is a model. She specializes in commercial camera studies of her face. Her face *is* her fortune, and her lovely eyes have looked out at you from national magazines many times in the past. In the terrible war to stay thin, that most models have, she developed an abdominal problem. It got worse. The first to show it were her eyes. At first they became dull and murky. Then they took on a

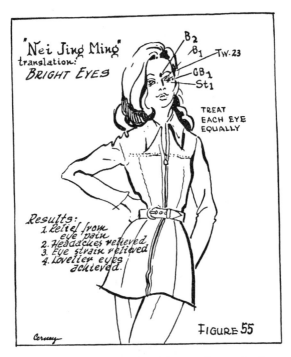

"Nei Jing Ming"
translation:
BRIGHT EYES

B2
B1 — TW.23
GB1
St1

TREAT
EACH EYE
EQUALLY

Results:
1. Relief from
   eye pain
2. Headaches relieved
3. Eye strain relieved
4. Lovelier eyes
   achieved.

FIGURE 55

yellowish cast shot with little red vessels, and those normally beautiful eyes were no longer pretty to look at. In closeup they were ghastly, and it was so devastating to Joanie that she thought her career was through.

Her New York physician put her in the hospital, but for some reason rest and medication didn't help. She came back home to our town.

Since I'd taken care of her since she was a little girl, she came in to see me. I told her about acupuncture and *Acupressure, U.S.A.* "Let's give it a whirl," she said, and we did. Two weeks later, Joanie was back in New York City, clear-eyed and happy. We used the procedure indicated above, put her on a bowel-cleansing diet, got her gall bladder working, and she's happily back in the camera's eye once more. Her lovely eyes will continue to stare at you from the nation's top magazines, and it was all done with *Acupressure, U.S.A.!*

Breast Beautification

Technique for Figure 56. In the breast-conscious United States, "It's what's up front that counts." So to develop more lovely breasts, apply palmar pressure in circular motions, with the fingertips cupped under the breast. Massaging gently, use a rotating motion, gently kneading each breast in such manner that the inside of the hand is cuplike at the bottom of the breast and the nipple is projecting through the aperture made by the thumb and index fingers.

With each rotation, use a lifting forward pressure. One beautiful blonde movie star used this method before stepping out on the sound stage. It was very uplifting to all concerned. The *Kidney, Stomach, Pericardium* and *Spleen meridians* are all involved in this process, and the stimulation of *Acupressure, U.S.A.* leads to achievement of the full-breastedness of youth once more.

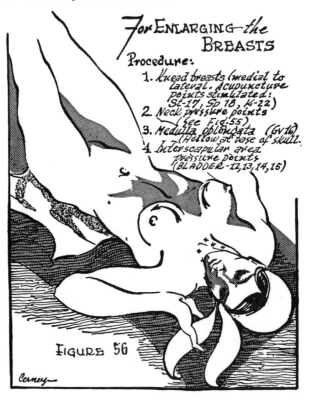

For ENLARGING the BREASTS

Procedure:
1. Knead breasts (medial to lateral. Acupuncture points stimulated: St-17, Sp 18, K-22)
2. Neck pressure points (see Fig. 55)
3. Medulla oblongata (GV 16) (Hollow at base of skull.
4. Interscapular area pressure points (BLADDER-12,13,14,15)

Figure 56

Cerney

Tension Release

Technique for Figure 57. The abnormal tensions of everyday life are age-makers today. They need release. You can release them by grasping the heavy muscles running from the skull down the neck to the shoulder. Grasp them between the thumb and other fingers. Compress at 1 inch intervals. Move from above down. Then pressure-massage downwardly on these muscles. As you do this, note the contractions or knots in these muscles. If a tension-spot is present, sink a fingertip into it. Hold till it dissolves beneath your fingertip. *Small Intestine meridian* point 15 is affected, as are *Triple Warmer* 15 and *Gall Bladder meridian* point 21.

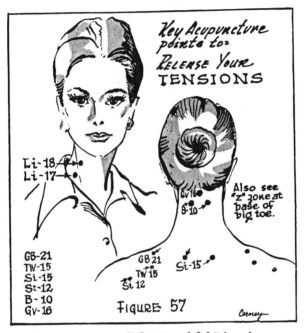

"Magic Buttons" for Youthful Digestion

Technique for Figure 58. Since food is one of the body's fuels, digestion must be maintained to preserve the factors of youth. To assist your digestion, here are those "magic buttons" to press, and how.

Cup the fingers of both hands under the right rib cage. The *Gall Bladder* and *Spleen meridians* are present in this area and GB-24 and Sp-16 are involved. Acupress! Hold for the three count. Release. Breathe deeply. Press inwardly once more. Hold. Exhale on the three count. Repeat five times.

Do the same over the gall bladder area on the right side of your abdomen at *Stomach meridian* acupuncture point 21. Then move to the solar plexus area. At Cv-14 and 15, repeat the same procedure.

Finish this series of actions with the fingers buried in the area of the umbilicus (Cv-8). Each area may be an area of hurt. Expect this in the beginning. Also know that as this discomfort eases up, those organs and meridians are less in conflict, digestion is taking place, cells are revitalizing, health is on its way.

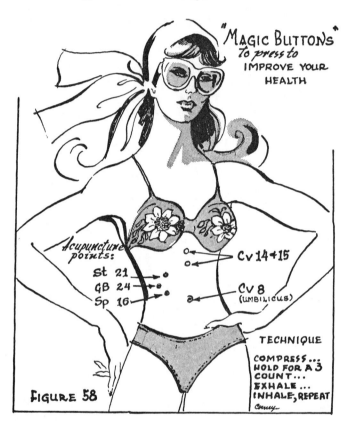

How to Step Up Vitality

Technique for Figure 59. Long hidden from this hemisphere have been many Oriental secrets. One of these secrets is that of maintaining youthful energy, and bringing a new glow to the face and new vitality to the body. To help you revitalize your body and your life, I want you to turn to an acupuncture point that traditional Chinese call *Ch'i Hai.* This is Conception Vessel acupuncture point 6 and is known as the "Sea of Ch'i" (or Q'i), otherwise known as the *Center of Energy!* Just below it is *Conception Vessel 5.* This is called

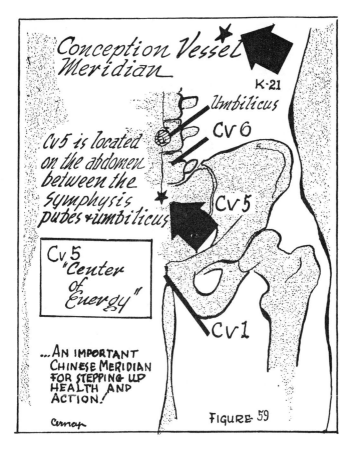

Conception Vessel Meridian

K-21

Umbilicus

Cv 6

Cv5 is located on the abdomen between the symphysis pubes + umbilicus

Cv 5

Cv 5 *"Center of Energy"*

Cv 1

...An important Chinese Meridian for stepping up health and action!

Carnay

Figure 59

Shi-Men. It too is a center of energy, and both lie conveniently accessible on the body's midline, just a few fingers below the umbilicus. Both influence the abdominal and pelvic contents where the youth forces lie.

Both are power sources when you need them most. Both stimulate the ovaries of the female and the testes of the male. Both increase sexual desire. Both help bring back to life those who have gone through mental and physical torture.

How well acupuncture points Cv-5 and 6 work are told in the story of Elaine D. Elaine was once a nun known as Sister Mary. While assigned to the Puerto Rican area of New York City, she fell in love with a social worker, a brilliant young man who worked by her side day after day. Sister Mary couldn't help it. She fell in love and lived in torture night and day, and because of it her body became a graveyard of physical destruction. Her loveliness disappeared. Her eyes no longer glowed. Her face sagged, and she pulled back deeper into her shroud of poor health. Her body cried out with the agony of wanting this young man, and yet her training forbade all this. She became sick. Her energy sapped away. She ended up in a wheelchair—and after throwing herself down the staircase twice, her Sister Superior confronted her.

Elaine obtained her freedom. When I saw her for the first time she was a mental and physical wreck, and the rehabilitation program seemed almost impossible. We went to work, and those first timid steps into the future of her physical and mental happiness began with the "SIX-POINT PROGRAM" that is in your hands at this moment. Step by step, we used Oriental techniques to achieve her desire.

In addition to office care, I helped Elaine choose such intimate little things as perfumes, hair-do's, and styles of clothing most advantageous to her figure. It was a long, hard row to hoe, but the day I put her on the plane to return to New York, I felt proud that I had helped her back to health. A few weeks later came an invitation. Elaine was to be married! Nine months later came another letter. Elaine had achieved the ultimate in womanhood. She had a baby—a boy—and it was named after me.

In this remarkable story, is the even more remarkable capability of the human being to recuperate, rehabilitate, and rejuvenate by using Chinese acupuncture points. It was one of the proudest days of my life when I saw Elaine D. getting on that plane for New York.

THE FOUNTAIN OF YOUTH
IS WITHIN YOU

Age is a state of mind long before it becomes a bodily condition. Anyone who would live longer and stay younger has to take advantage of Nature. Chronologically the years may pile up in the body, but not in the brain, and to revive glandular vitality and help yourself in health, beauty, and go-power, you have to use your head about *Acupressure, U.S.A.*

If You're Past 30 Years Old,
Rejuvenation Begins Now!

In using your head with *Acupressure, U.S.A.*, start by forgetting your chronological years. Wash the count out of your mind. I'm not asking you to think young. What I am saying is that you are as old as you make yourself feel, so why not make yourself feel younger?

"Think not ye old," said our minister from his rostrum a short time back, and all around me I saw backs straightening. It was mind over matter. In my mind, as I listened to the sermon, I was saying, "And don't forget to tell them about acupuncture points to keep them from getting old," but he never did. His idea was to "think young," and this of course is a good, positive approach, but it takes something even more. It takes getting those fountains of youth within you to work.

Aging comes from neglect and failure. Aging is what shows when one or more physiological links begin to weaken because you're not keeping them under control. You're not using the fountains of youth within you.

No matter how young you are, you are already old when you can no longer bend and touch the floor. When you have difficulty getting up out of a chair, when keenness of mind slips away, when wrinkles and fat pads begin to show, when the skin of your elbows gets rough, when jowls hang, and when a fold of skin caught between two fingers is thicker than a quarter inch, you are already growing old. Each one of these signposts is an alarm, signalling neglect. Because of this, rejuvenation is a personal matter. It's the failure to use the natural powers within yourself. The Chinese had the answers to this. They stimulated endocrine glands, used mental control, mind over matter, and got results.

Acupressure, the Answer to Problems of Aging

The Orientals *do* have answers to the process of aging, via acupuncture and acupressure, and by dealing directly with acupuncture points, you can re-activate your endocrine glands (testes, ovaries, adrenals, pituitary, thyroid, etc.). Through acupuncture points, you can revive glandular activity and restore function. Through acupuncture points, you can regenerate new cellular growth, and new cells of youth are begun again. If you have the desire—if you have the will—to rejuvenate and recuperate, you can set this fountain of youth to flowing once more.

HOW TO REJUVENATE THE FACE

A B C SCHEDULE OF ACTION

A	B	C	D	E	F	G
Si-17	St-4	B-2	Li-4	Liv-14	GB-20	Ball of Big Toe

Explanation of Contact Points

(A) At angle of jaw (behind and below) (Si-17).

(B) At corners of mouth (S-4).

(C) At nose side of each eye brow (B-2).

(D) Dorsum of hand, first and second metacarpals, form a web (Li-4).

(E) Rib cage (third from the bottom) (Liv-14).

(F) At the base of the skull, just behind the mastoid process (GB-20).

(G) Ball of big toe (reflex point massage). (Massage all other reflex pain points on the bottom of the foot and above the ankle.)

PROBLEMS OF THE EYES AND HOW TO COPE WITH THEM

Although many problems assail the eyes, I am going to deal primarily with three simple ones with which you may readily cope. Such factors as *conjunctivitis, styes,* and *blepharitis* will be dealt with here. The reason for doing this is because of the very importance of sight itself and the need for professional help.

When eye problems occur, consult your oculist, your ophthalmologist, or optometrist. He will check for visual acuity with and without glasses. He will determine how the ocular muscles are working. Margins and subcutaneous tissues will be examined. Lacrimal sacs will be investigated. A tonometer will be used to determine ocular tension. Size and shape of the pupils and their reactions to light and accommodation are recorded. Your eye doctor will also look inside the eye. He will use an ophthalmoscope to bring the retina into focus. The retina, behind the open iris, is a tattletale.

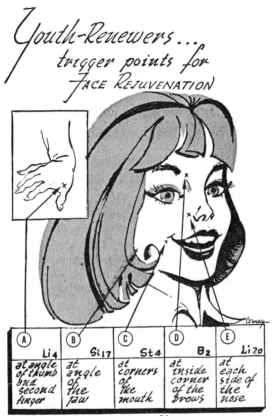

Youth-Renewers...
trigger points for
Face Rejuvenation

Ⓐ	Ⓑ	Ⓒ	Ⓓ	Ⓔ
Li 4	Si 17	St 4	B 2	Li 20
at angle of thumb and second finger	at angle of the jaw	at corners of the mouth	at inside corner of the brows	at each side of the nose

FIGURE 60

It's a tattletale because it shows blood vessel change. It mirrors systemic diseases such as nephritis, high blood pressure, and diabetes. Your doctor will use slit lamps and other instrumentation to determine whether you actually have an eye problem. In case of direct injury, he determines the tissues involved and the reparative course to follow. All such complex problems should be left in his hands. He knows a lot more about it than you do. Of the three conditions mentioned earlier, an answer lies in *acupuncture without needles.*

Conjunctivitis

Conjunctivitis is simply an inflammation of the mucous membrane lining the eyelids.

In down-to-earth language, conjunctivitis is called *"pink-eye."* Dust, smoke, bright lights, wind, reflection on snow or water or ice may cause it. Bacteria may be the offending agent. Usually it starts with the eyes watering. Both eyelids begin to itch and burn. The conjunctiva and corners of the eyes become bright red. Swelling of the lids and purulence may occur, sealing the lids shut. Sometimes this lasts for a number of days. In other cases, it may last for weeks. Luckily, it is self-limiting. However, you may hasten its demise—or even prevent it—by prompt acupressure therapy.

A B C SCHEDULE OF ACTION

A	B	C	D	E	F
Tw-23	GB-20	St-8 44	B-1	Gv-16	L-1

(See explanation of contact points)

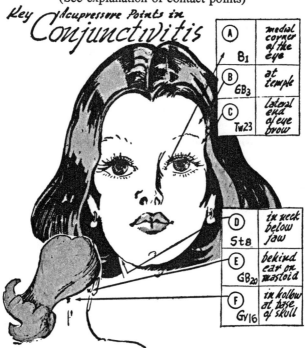

Key Acupressure Points in
Conjunctivitis

(A) B1	medial corner of the eye
(B) GB3	at temple
(C) Tw23	lateral end of eye brow
(D) St8	in neck below jaw
(E) GB20	behind ear on mastoid
(F) Gv16	in hollow at base of skull

FIGURE 61

**Explanation of
Contact Points**

(A) Outside end of eye brows (Tw-23).

(B) GB-1 is located at the lateral end of each eye brow. GB-3 is found in the temples above the jaw hinge. GB-20 is found at the base of the skull.

(C) St-8 may be located just below each jaw. St-44 is located at the base (dorsally) of the second toe.

(D) Liv-2 is located at the first joint on the lateral side of the great toe.

(E) B-1 is found at the inner corner of the eye.

(F) Gv-16 is located midline on the spine where skull sits on the first cervical vertebra.

**Supplementary
Procedures**

1. *Prophylactic treatment*
   a. Cold, damp cloths on the eyes.
   b. Wear dark glasses.
   c. Avoid dust, wind, sun, smoke, bright light.
   d. Don't rub your eyes!
   e. Relax.
   f. Get more sleep.
   g. Regulate your diet (add fruit and vegetables—fresh—and cut down on meat and potatoes and candy and pastry).

Styes

Styes are circumscribed inflammations of sebaceous glands in or near the edge of an eyelid, creating a condition which may or may not terminate in suppuration (pus, etc.).

Selma P. told me her family doctor said she had *hordeolum,* and since her parents didn't know what the word meant, they thought she was going to lose her eye. In everyday language, *hordeolum* is a stye. It's a local problem involving the meibomian glands in the eyelids and is usually due to invasion by some pus-forming bacteria (staphylococcus). Styes, however, may also be caused by general health, debility, a focus of infection somewhere in the body, neck, or head, or even "bad eyes" that need glasses. Selma said that her stye began by feeling like she "had something in her eye." Everybody insisted on looking. Nobody saw anything. That also applied to her family doctor, because in the beginning stages nothing tangible is obvious. The lids and the eye then become red and begin to water. Following this stage comes swelling and a small, round, red, tender area on the lid that turns into a suppurating abscess. She said that as soon as the stye ruptured, she experienced relief from the problem. This same problem may graduate or progress to *blepharitis* or a *chalazion*.

A B C SCHEDULE OF ACTION

A	B	C	D	E	F
B-1	GB-1	T-17	Si-7	L-11	St-44

**Explanation of
Contact Points**

(A) Medial corner of each eye (B-1).

(B) GB-1 is at the lateral end of each eye.

(C) Behind ear, on neck, at level of mastoid process for Tw-17.

(D) Eight finger widths up from the lateral side of the wrist for Si-7.

(E) Thumb, at level of nail root, for L-11.

(F) St-44 may be located at point where toes two and three meet the foot.

**Supplementary
Procedures**

1. *Physical therapy.*

a. Cold toweling over the eyes (*no ice!*). This relieves congestion, itching, and hurt. When suppuration comes to a head, use hot wetpacks.

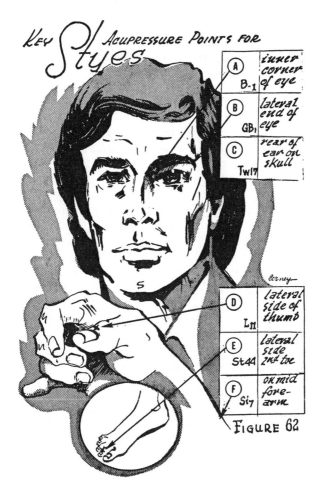

Key Acupressure Points for Styes

A	B-1	inner corner of eye
B	GB₁	lateral end of eye
C	Tw17	rear of ear on skull
D	L₁₁	lateral side of thumb
E	St44	lateral side 2nd toe
F	Si7	on mid fore-arm

FIGURE 62

2. *Determine whether you have an infection.*

More often than not, there is an infection somewhere in the neck, head, or body when a stye occurs. Like an acupuncture point pain area, a stye must occur on the eye and its cause is far removed.

3. *Prophylaxis.*

    a. Stop using your eyes so much.

    b. Relax! Take it easy around the clock for awhile.

    c. Add Vitamins A and D to your diet. Eat plenty of fresh fruit and vegetables.

d. If a stye is persistent, see your family physician. He may use an autogenous vaccine. However, if you use your acupuncture trigger points effectively, you may never have a re-occurrence of styes again.

Blepharitis

Blepharitis is an inflammation of the eyelid complicated by swelling, possible ulceration, and the formation of crusts and scales.

When I first saw Grace McG., her eyelash follicles were red and inflammation was creeping around the rims. An allergy had set the problem going. In other people, the resistance being down gives infection an entrée. Poor diet may precipitate the problem, and in its wake come the redness noticed so quickly, the burning, watering of the eye, and itching. As this continues, the lashes tend to fall out. The eyeball also gets involved. The eye fights light. Shallow ulcers form in the lids and exude fluid that gets crusty and glues the eyelids shut during the night. The problem is annoying and recurrent and doesn't respond too well to treatment of normal procedure. Not so with *Acupressure, U.S.A.* It's faster and more efficient. Here's how it's done.

A B C SCHEDULE OF ACTION

A	B	C	D	E	F	G	H	I	J
1 B-2	1 GB-3 18 20	10 Cv-13	2 Li-4	L-5	S-43	Si-4	S-36	T-10	H-3

Explanation of
Contact Points

(A) B-1 is located at the inner corner of each eye. B-2 is found at the inside end of each brow.

(B) GB-1 is at the outside corner of each eye, GB-3 in the temple just above each jaw bone joint. GB-18 is on the skull four finger widths above the ear, and GB-20 is on the back of the neck two finger widths from the mastoid process (toward center line).

(C) Cv-10 is found on the spinal midline between the processes of lumbar vertebrae 2 and 3. Cv-13 is at joint level between thoracic vertebrae 9 and 10.

(D) In the web between index finger and thumb is Li-4. Li-2 is on the thumb side of the index finger at its third joint.

(E) Just in front of the elbow is L-5.

(F) Where the second and third toes meet the foot is St-43.

(G) Si-4 is at the lateral border of the hand.

(H) St-36 is located approximately four finger widths below the knee cap on the outside of the leg.

(I) Slightly above the elbow's "crazy bone" and behind the elbow is Tw-10.

(J) On the body side of each elbow is H-3.

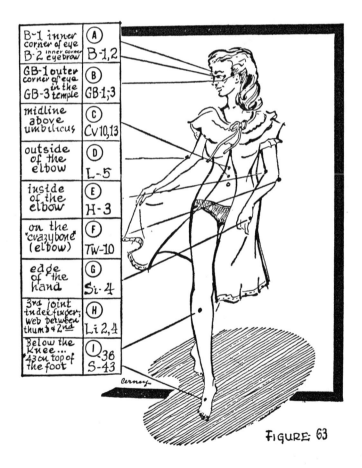

B-1 inner corner of eye B-2 inner corner eyebrow	(A)	B-1,2
GB-1 outer corner of eye GB-3 temple in the	(B)	GB-1;3
midline above umbilicus	(C)	Cv 10,13
outside of the elbow	(D)	L-5
inside of the elbow	(E)	H-3
on the "crazybone" (elbow)	(F)	Tw-10
edge of the hand	(G)	Si-4
3rd joint index finger; web between thumb & 2nd	(H)	Li 2,4
Below the knee... 43 on top of the foot	(I)	36 S-43

FIGURE 63

GENERAL EYE CONDITIONS

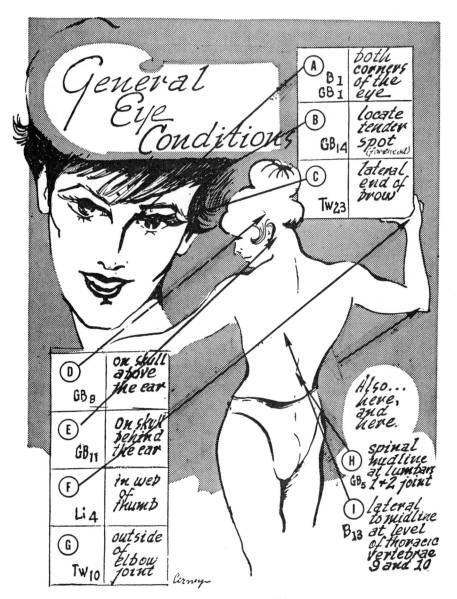

Ⓐ	B₁ GB₁	both corners of the eye
Ⓑ	GB₁₄	locate tender spot (forehead)
Ⓒ	Tw₂₃	lateral end of brow
Ⓓ	GB₈	on skull above the ear
Ⓔ	GB₁₁	on skull behind the ear
Ⓕ	Li₄	in web of thumb
Ⓖ	Tw₁₀	outside of elbow joint

Also... here, and here.

Ⓗ	GB₅	spinal midline at lumbar 1+2 joint
Ⓘ	B₁₃	lateral to midline at level of thoracic vertebrae 9 and 10

FIGURE 64

THE EARS

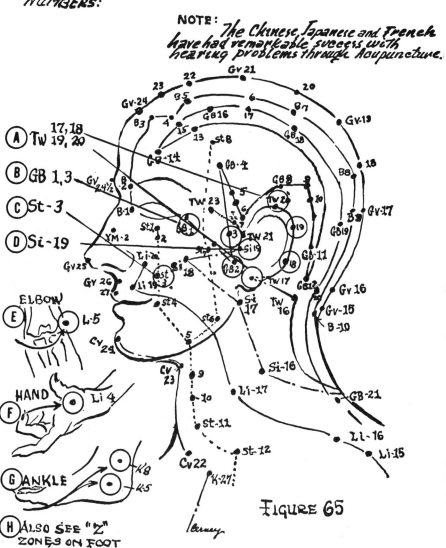

Acupress ONLY the CIRCLED NUMBERS:

DEAFNESS

NOTE: *The Chinese, Japanese and French have had remarkable success with hearing problems through Acupuncture.*

(A) Tw 17, 18, 19, 20

(B) GB 1, 3

(C) St-3

(D) Si-19

(E) ELBOW — L-5

(F) HAND — Li 4

(G) ANKLE — K 8, K 5

(H) ALSO SEE "Z" ZONES ON FOOT

FIGURE 65

Deafness

A Musician Has His
Hearing Restored

Johnny V. played lead guitar with one of those modern combinations of electronic noise-makers. They not only entertained but also maintained a guaranteed noise-level. After high school, Johnny left the amateurs, bought an even higher volume electronic guitar, and hit the road. By the time he was 21, he couldn't hear normal conversation. When he finally came home, the loss of hearing was his big complaint. Upon examination, I found his ear drums sclerosed. By way of his ears, he was already an old man, a guitar-type Beethoven without the same kind of talent. I recommended an ear surgeon and the tube-transplant failed. Johnny still couldn't hear, so I recommended *Acupressure, U.S.A.* He wanted to know more about it. I told him about the British physician Felix Mann who cured 66% of such problems, how the Chinese physicians were showing an even higher percentage of cures, and the Russians were doing the same. I went on to tell him about other reasons for hearing loss.

The causes for loss of hearing are many. Changes take place in the ear drum, middle ear, external auditory canal, the nerves and blood vessels, and even the eustachian tubes. Hearing loss may have its inception in the sensory area of the brain. Foreign bodies may also play a role. Mechanical obstructions to hearing may be due to wax, beans, peas, or bugs. Deafness may follow treatment by streptomycin or come to the female after menopause sets in. There may be boils in the ears, perforations, or scarring. The ossicles may harden. There may be damage to the eighth cranial or auditory nerve, to the auditory center, or to the cerebral nerves carrying the messages in and out of the brain. Any or all of these complex structures may be involved by infectious disease. They may be involved by overdosages of such toxic wastes as alcohol, salicylates, arsenic, or quinine. All very complicated, and it takes a little doing to conquer it! It took a little doing with Johnny, and here are the acupuncture points we used for successful results.

Tinnitus

Definition: Tinnitus is a tinkling, ringing, or other kind of sound heard only by the person, and is caused by conditions of the external, middle, and inside ear. Noises in *tinnitus* may range from roaring and whistling to buzzing and bumpety-bumping. It may be off-again, on-again or constant. The person who has it may be told by his doctor that it is caused by hardening of the arteries, high blood pressure, or even heavy drug ingestion. Tooth and jaw problems may excite it. Endocrine glands may contribute to the problem. Hysteria may play a role. Something so simple as impacted ear wax may set it off. Churchman Martin Luther was one of those who heard sounds in his head (tinnitus cerebri). He had Meniere's disease, and on the basis of sounds in his head which he attributed to the devil, he promulgated a religion. For a technic to alleviate these foreign "sounds," following is the *Acupressure, U.S.A.* approach to use. See Figure 66.

A B C SCHEDULE OF ACTION

A	B	C
Tw-17, 18 19, 20	Si-19	GB-1 2

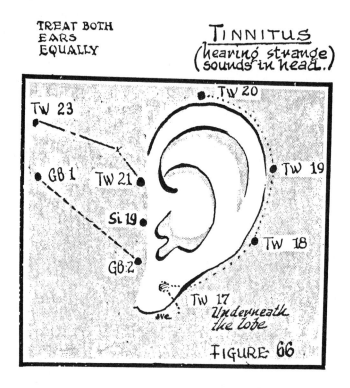

TREAT BOTH EARS EQUALLY

TINNITUS
(hearing strange sounds in head.)

FIGURE 66

THE HUMAN MOUTH

A few Chinese terms for mouth conditions that can be treated with acupressure and acupuncture are *Kou Mi, Kou Chuang,* and *E*

Kou Chuang. Keenly aware of the necessity for proper diagnosis of health problems, traditional Chinese acupuncturists wrapped up each problem in tidy packages before giving it a name and treatment procedure. Today we have the outcome of their meticulous research findings. Thousands of years ago, they were already ahead of the 20th Century. They had something that we in the United States are just beginning to recognize and see. Just how effectively acupuncture and acupressure can be may be noted in the following procedures for *gingivitis, toothache, dry mouth,* and *coughing,* each a procedure that can be applied at home.

Gingivitis

Gingivitis is an inflammation and swelling of the gums, accompanied by congestion and bleeding on pressure, or while brushing the teeth, but demonstrating no significant pain.

There are many reasons why the gums may swell and bleed, and they are not due to conditions of the teeth. Gingivitis may be due to a too stiff bristle on your toothbrush, or to the use of strong mouthwashes. It may be due to the teeth and jaws being out-of-line, improper chewing habits, food impactions, faulty false teeth, mouth breathing, and even dental "bridges" and other metalwork that spell out trouble. Your family doctor, or dentist, may have to check even more deeply if gingivitis continues. In my own practice, I have found that gingivitis presents itself as an initial symptom in systemic disorders. It may be due to a lack of vitamins in the diet. It may be due to diabetes, drug ingestion, glandular disturbances, or even to allergies.

When Lorrie Layne C. presented herself for physical examination for insurance, she asked about the red band at her gum line. It was simply a red line along the edge of the teeth. She said it wasn't sensitive but that it bled easily. I found her gums engorged, edematous, and rose-red in color. Some of the gum line was drawn back, exposing the roots of a few teeth that were actually loose in their sockets. Her tongue was bright red and smooth; her lips red and cracked. She said her mouth felt like it was scalded, and she was afraid to kiss her beau. Lorrie Layne, like many others in opulent U.S.A. living the beautiful life, was one of those starving to death in the midst of plenty. What did she have? Through poor eating habits she had *pellagra,* a severe Vitamin B deficiency, and *Acupressure, U.S.A.* is a procedure of choice in coping with gingivitis due to this dietary problem. Here's the Chinese approach. See Figure 67.

A B C SCHEDULE OF ACTION

A	B	C	D	E	F
Gv-28	GB-16	Tw-17	St-4	Si-4	Li-4

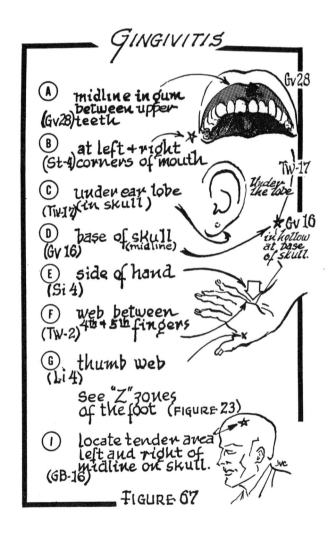

GINGIVITIS

(A) midline in gum between upper (Gv28) teeth

Gv 28

(B) at left + right (St-4) corners of mouth

(C) under ear lobe (Tw-17) (in skull)

Tw-17
Under the lobe

(D) base of skull (midline) (Gv 16)

★ Gv 16
in hollow at base of skull.

(E) side of hand (Si 4)

(F) web between 4th + 5th fingers (TW-2)

(G) thumb web (Li 4)

See "Z" zones of the foot (FIGURE 23)

(I) locate tender area left and right of midline on skull. (GB-16)

FIGURE 67

Supplementary
Procedures

1. *Niacinamide* (at least 5 mgs per day).
2. Completely balanced and wholesome meals.
3. Plenty of sleep.
4. Improved health habits.

Toothache

Toothache is that neuralgic pain resulting from irritation, infection, and/or inflammation of the dental pulp.

A tooth is not bone. It is made up of dentine encased in cement and covered with white enamel. Its crown remains exposed. Its roots are buried in the jaw, and through these roots blood vessels and nerves find entrance. Too often, because of pain in a local area, teeth are removed. Too often these teeth are demonstrated to have no actual problem. They were not involved. What *was* involved was the nervous system and a referred pain to the part. When the electronic forces of pain collect in a given area, they must be shunted away, and this is why acupuncture and *Acupressure, U.S.A.* are so valuable in mouth care. To help you on this score, here are the emergency acupuncture points involved. See Figure 68.

A B C SCHEDULE OF ACTION

A	B	C	D	E
6 St-28 44	2 GB-17 37	Li-4 6	Tw-21	B-69

Supplementary   (See Figure 68)
Procedures

1. *Physical therapy.*
   a. Ice rub on pressure points.
   b. Additional acupuncture points to treat:
      Temple pressure

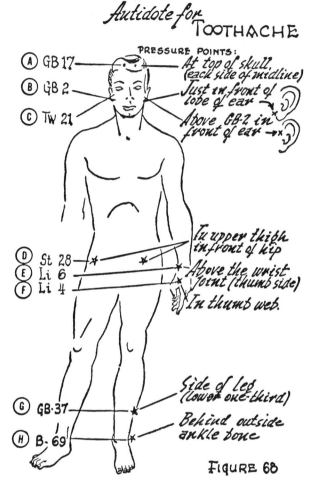

Antidote for TOOTHACHE

PRESSURE POINTS:

Ⓐ GB 17 — *At top of skull, (each side of midline)*

Ⓑ GB 2 — *Just in front of lobe of ear*

Ⓒ TW 21 — *Above GB-2 in front of ear*

Ⓓ St 28 — *In upper thigh in front of hip*

Ⓔ Li 6 — *Above the wrist joint (thumb side)*

Ⓕ Li 4 — *In thumb web.*

Ⓖ GB-37 — *Side of leg (lower one-third)*

Ⓗ B. 69 — *Behind outside ankle bone*

FIGURE 68

Apply three fingers on the temple on the side of the toothache. Press. Release. Hold. Repeat at least five times for pressure on Tw-22 and GB-7.

Jaw pressure

Apply three-finger pressure (hold without release for a 50 count) on the jaw involved.

Fingertip pressure above or below the aching tooth (determined by upper or lower jaw).
Carotid artery pressure

This procedure must be gently diplomatic. NOTE: apply pressure on the carotid artery *only*, on the side of the aching tooth. Be gentle but firm. Hold for the three count and release. Repeat three times.

2. *Oil of cloves.*
This is an old Chinese remedy if acupressure does not give you immediate results.

Dry Mouth

Dry mouth is that condition in which there is a complete lack of saliva (aptyalism) in the mouth.

Carrie had "dry mouth." Carrie is an older woman whom nobody tells what to do . . . and this includes doctors. She doesn't listen to instruction, advice, or other conversation. She knows more than anyone else in the whole wide world, and you know people just like her. Then came some personal shocks, like her husband dying and her daughter getting killed and her son a missing person in the Vietnam war. She couldn't be blamed for her current state of mind under those circumstances, and I maintained silence as I examined the problem for which a relative of hers had brought her into my office.

I noted that her tongue was like crocodile hide—cracked, rough, thick. She said her teeth had actually "dropped out" and that she had no sense of taste. Since she was a close relative of one of my Tennessee friends who brought her to our town for therapy, I had to advise her about how she could use *Acupressure, U.S.A.* on herself. I told her that her problem was called "dry mouth," and she said, "It sure is. I can't spit good." We rendered treatment at the office and gave her written instructions to follow. Not long afterward, I received a telephone call from Carrie's relative. He said, "Aunt Carrie's sure OK. She can spit farther than any of us now."

A B C SCHEDULE OF ACTION

A	B	C
Gv-28	Liv-8	L-5

Chinese Acupressure Points for DRY MOUTH

3 KEY CONTACTS

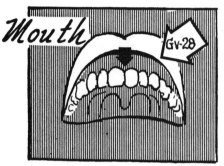

Mouth

GV-28

(A) GV-28

Make first contact on midline between teeth (upper)

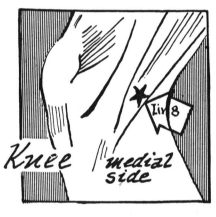

Knee   medial side

Liv 8

(B) LIV-8

Locate tenderness zone. Treat.

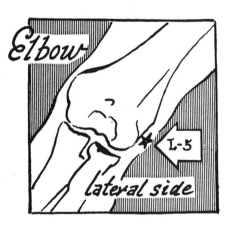

Elbow

L-5

lateral side

(C) L-5

Use rotary pressure-technique for results.

FIGURE 69

**Supplementary
Procedures**

1. *Better-fitting dentures.*
2. *Dietary balance.* Add Vitamins A, C, E, and B Complex to mineral supplements.
3. *Glycerin mouthwash.*

Coughing

Coughing is any forceful expiration of air in an effort to relieve the throat. Coughing has many causes. It may be dry. It may be moist. It may be productive or non-productive, as far as bringing up phlegm is concerned. It may be the result of asthma, heart problems, or from the bronchial tubes. It may stem from the larynx or swelling of the thyroid. There's a cough present in pneumonia and diphtheria, a reflex cough in the whooping of pertussis. All these coughs begin with a local irritant. Whether it be the "common cold," measles, or pharyngitis, a cough is a symptom that all have in common.

A family in our neighborhood had a rather frightening experience with their Johnny. Johnny was aged ten. He was a smart child, reading college textbooks while still in grammar school. His family simply couldn't cope with his brilliance. The only time he became other than a "brain" was when his coughing spells set in. Then he became a kid again and put his head on Mommy's breast and snuggled close for security.

As a neighborhood practitioner I'd heard about Johnny's coughing spells, but I'd never seen the boy until he'd made the rounds of specialists. In making my study of the lad, when finally they brought him in, I was thinking about those two Chinese words *Ke Sou* which means "couch." The literature of Fianshi records *Ke Sou* as "empty lung." In this boy, there was a shortness of breath. Just a short walk brought on difficulty in breathing. He had a dry mouth and complained of his throat being parched. He was *shen* weary. His voice was weak and low, his face white. His skin was dry, almost withered. His pulse had an empty feel. With this in mind I began—and successfully brought to a halt—the coughing brought on by these conditions. Following is the *Acupressure, U.S.A.* techniques I used. Within a few days, his cough was gone.

A B C SCHEDULE OF ACTION

A	B	C	D
Cv-6 12	B-37 38	St-36	L-1

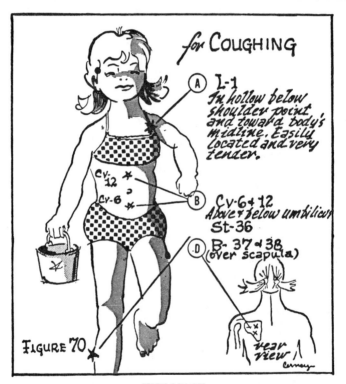

for COUGHING

Ⓐ L-1
In hollow below shoulder point and toward body's midline. Easily located and very tender.

Cv-12
Cv-6

Ⓑ Cv-6 + 12
Above + below umbilicus
St-36

Ⓓ B-37 + 38
(over scapula)

rear view

FIGURE 70

THE NOSE

Nose Bleed

Nose bleed is any hemorrhage from the nostrils.

The medical term for the condition is "epistaxis." Nose bleed may have many causes. It may be due to bone fracture, nose picking, foreign bodies, allergies, tumors, sinusitis, or a blow to the head. It may come as the result of a systemic disease. Hypertension (high blood pressure), hardening of the arteries, or kidney problems may bring it on. Stepping out of an air-conditioned office into the heat of a summer day may precipitate it. If epistaxis continues, your doctor is the best one to determine the cause and the therapy necessary. Acupuncture points to use to advantage in the interim are as follows. You may never have to see a doctor on this matter again. See Figure 71.

A B C SCHEDULE OF ACTION

A	B	C	D	E	F	G	H
L-5	Liv-5	Si-2 7	B-10 18	Li-4 10 11 19 20	Gv-14 15 16 20 21 24	P-8	GB-12

(Consult other illustrations for above "points")

Supplementary Procedures

1. *Physical therapy.*
   a. Pack involved side of nose with 1-inch gauze.
   b. Place coldpack over bridge of nose and at nape of neck.
   c. Sit upright, head backward.
   d. Place thumb in hollow at base of skull. Apply pressure with thumb forwardly as you use the other hand on the forehead to bring the head backwardly. Massage the area (direct influence on the medulla oblongata) until bleeding stops. NOTE: Quite often this is the only pressure point you need. The Chinese label this as *Governing Vessel meridian* point 16.

Sinusitis

Sinusitis is any inflammation of a sinus chamber, with accessory sinuses becoming involved. See Figure 72.

A catarrhal problem may develop in the inner lining of the sinus chambers at any time. When the inflammation from this non-health problem takes place, there will also be inflammation in the nose. In acute suppurative sinusitis there may be purulent inflammation, with such symptoms as headache, chills, fever, and pain over the sinus directly involved. Treatment should remain conservative until otherwise proven wrong.

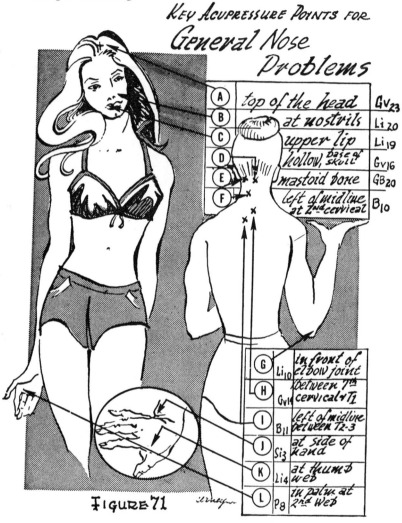

KEY ACUPRESSURE POINTS FOR

General Nose Problems

Ⓐ	top of the head	GV23
Ⓑ	at nostrils	Li20
Ⓒ	upper lip	Li19
Ⓓ	hollow, base of skull	GV16
Ⓔ	mastoid bone	GB20
Ⓕ	left of midline at 2nd cervical	B10

Ⓖ	Li10	in front of elbow joint
Ⓗ	GV14	between 7th cervical + T1
Ⓘ	B11	left of midline between T2-3
Ⓙ	Si3	at side of hand
Ⓚ	Li4	at thumb web
Ⓛ	P8	in palm at 2nd web

FIGURE 71

When I was boxing, I got clobbered often enough. Blows to the head are one reason for sinus involvement. The result was that I had a deviated septum. The turbinates enlarged. The sinuses failed to drain. My sparring partner, Jodie F., had the same thing. Jodie weighed in at 150, moved like a panther, and was totally efficient until his nose got hit. Putting his nose on target gave him more than a sore nose. Inflamed sinuses resulted in headaches, pain, discharge, and dizziness. Sometimes the pain was so bad that even his teeth hurt. When this happened, he couldn't even go for three fast rounds of sparring practice.

Some folks may have acute sinusitis from rhinitis (inflammation of the nasal lining). Some may get it from allergies or even from emotional upsets. One case that baffled me for a while was a lovely little girl with a thick, purulent discharge coming from her nose in a never ending flow. Inside, when once it was cleaned sufficiently to see, the nasal mucosa (inner lining) was boggy, red, and thick. The transilluminator up her nose failed to show through in the darkness of the examining room. X-ray views of her sinuses came up with an answer. Revealed was a small metal ball. A surgeon removed it. Cathy admitted inserting the lead pellet from her brother's BB gun. Following surgery, she was rendered the following Chinese approach to relieve the inflammation and congestion that was present.

A B C SCHEDULE OF ACTION

A	B	C	D	E	F
K-8	Liv-8	Gv-26 28 16	St-1 18	S-1 3 7 40 45	B-2 64

(Consult other illustrations such as Figure 65 for above "points")

Supplementary
Procedures

1. *Physical therapy.*
    a. Rinse inside of nose with salt water (1 tablespoonful salt to 1 quart of water).
    b. Coldpacks over bridge of nose and nape of neck.
2. *Dietary supplements.*
    a. Fresh fruits and green vegetables.
    b. Vitamin A (100,000 units daily for a week). Also add Vitamin C (*not* ascorbic acid!). It must be organically derived.
3. *Rest in bed.*
4. *Drink large quantity of water,* fruit, or vegetable juices.
5. *Additional pressure procedures* for sinusitis.

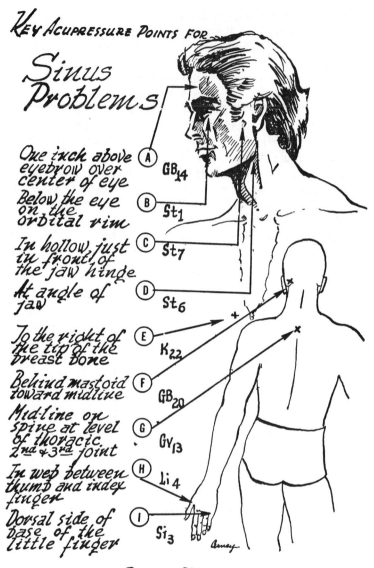

KEY ACUPRESSURE POINTS FOR

Sinus Problems

One inch above eyebrow over center of eye — (A) GB₁₄

Below the eye on the orbital rim — (B) St₁

In hollow, just in front of the jaw hinge — (C) St₇

At angle of jaw — (D) St₆

To the right of the tip of the breast bone — (E) K₂₂

Behind mastoid toward midline — (F) GB₂₀

Mid-line on spine at level of thoracic 2nd & 3rd joint — (G) Gv₁₃

In web between thumb and index finger — (H) Li 4

Dorsal side of base of the little finger — (I) Si₃

FIGURE 72

Technique

1. *Compress nose between index finger and thumb,* from bridge to tip of nose. Move downwardly to easy stages, compressing and releasing to the three count.

2. *Three-finger pressure on the forehead.* In a perpendicular line, place the fingertips of one hand up from the nose and compress. Follow this with three-finger compression over each eye.

3. *Temporal compression.* Place index fingertip in temple area. Search for spot that hurts. Compress this local area of pain off and on and off till gone.

4. *Jaw-hinge joint compression.* Locate the spot between the hinge of the jaw and the lobe of the ear. This area, in sinus problems, will often be exquisitely tender. Compress gently three times, with progressively stronger pressure.

5. *Thoracic pressure points.* Lean your weight back against a doorframe. Move your feet forward as you thrust your weight backward between the shoulder blade and the spinal column. Locate the most "ouchy" spot and hold. Then go to the other side of the spinal column. Repeat.

6. *Medulla oblongata area pressure.* Follow all therapy with the general shotgun of pressure on the medulla oblongata area! By so doing, you step up the functions of the autonomic system. This results in everything improving faster.

BONUS THERAPIES

The following illustrations and ABC Schedules of Action are for techniques not yet totally established. They *are*, however, on matters that crop up in a family time after time, such as:

(a) *Hayfever.*
(b) *Hiccoughing.*

EDITOR'S NOTE: The two therapies that follow are all in the experimental stage. The author has achieved modest success with each, but as yet cannot report consistent "cures." Do your own experimenting with a therapy from which there can be no detrimental after-effects. If you get no results, simply go to your physician.

What is presented here, in these "bonus therapies," is simply an Americanization—without needles—of acupuncture procedures that have been used for thousands of years . . . and a record, thousands of years old, is pretty hard to beat. "If it works, don't knock it," said one famous statesman, and it's just possible that *Acupressure, U.S.A.* may very well work for *you*!

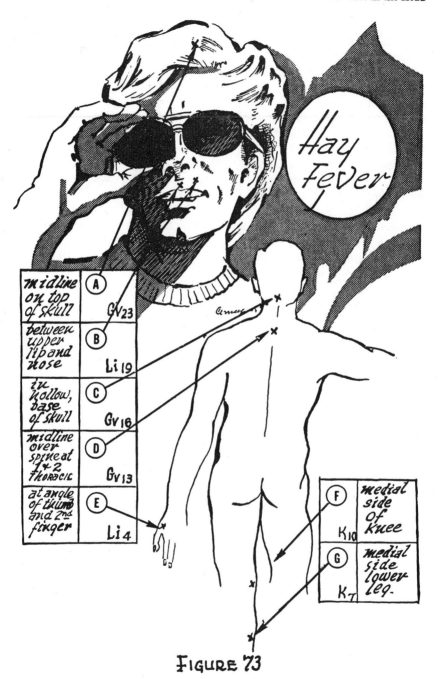

Hay Fever

midline on top of skull	(A)	GV23
between upper lip and nose	(B)	Li 19
in hollow, base of skull	(C)	GV 16
midline over spine at 1 & 2 thoracic	(D)	GV 13
at angle of thumb and 2nd finger	(E)	Li 4

(F)	medial side of knee
K10	
(G)	medial side lower leg.
K7	

FIGURE 73

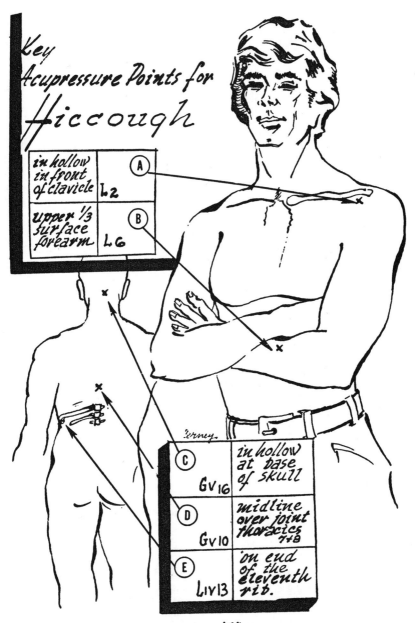

Key
Acupressure Points for
Hiccough

| in hollow in front of clavicle | L 2 | Ⓐ |
| upper ⅓ surface forearm | L 6 | Ⓑ |

Ⓒ	GV 16	in hollow at base of skull
Ⓓ	GV 10	midline over joint thoracics 7+8
Ⓔ	LIV 13	on end of the eleventh rib.

FIGURE 74

HOW TO HANDLE
AILMENTS OF THE NECK

5

Following are acupressure techniques for:

>"Crick" in neck
>Blood pressure problems
>Goiter and other thyroid problems
>Laryngitis
>Pharyngitis
>Swollen throat
>Tonsillitis
>Torticollis
>>Whiplash injury and "wry neck"

Also there are additional therapies for:

>Inability to bend head back
>Pain in neck or throat
>Sore throat (of unknown origin) or child's persistent cough
>Stiff neck
>Tension

BLOOD PRESSURE
AND NECK CONTROL POINTS
TO USE IN ACUPRESSURE, U.S.A.

Too much ado is made over "blood pressure" and too often people get a wrong concept about high and low blood pressure from neighbors, friends, all-knowing relatives, and sometimes doctors too. However, where low blood pressure, for example, *does* exist for any reason, it has to be established for what it is, and its cause determined, to get back to normal once more.

Low Blood Pressure
and Its Symptoms

How do you know when you have low blood pressure without a sphygmomanometer at hand? Some people never know. Others with low B/P may have dizziness. Their eyes may tire easily. They may be tired all the time, have headaches, and for some reason just can't seem to concentrate. They may have a tight feeling in their chest and their heart may palpitate. They have very little go-power and are among those who are the first to poop out. None of these symptoms are strong, but they spell out trouble in the future. They are warning signs to which you have to pay heed. How can *Acupressure, U.S.A.* be used to control the problem? Start with that neck control point called the "carotid sinus." It's Oriental magic!

Carotid Sinus

The carotid sinus is said to be a ductless gland. It is found at the bifurcation of the common carotid artery on either side of the neck and is easily accessible for *Acupressure, U.S.A.* Here's what you do:

Step One: Locate this enlargement on the internal carotid artery. (See Figure 75.) For a quickie landmark, locate the top of your Adam's apple and slide your finger back till you feel a pulsation. You're on the button! This very important gland regulates the blood pressure. It is attached to very special nerve-end-organs that have the ability to raise and lower blood pressure by way of a reflex arc over the carotid branch of the glossopharyngeal nerve. This stimulus is conveyed to that all-important medulla oblongata which increases or decreases the heart rate on demand. Press the carotid sinus. Then go to the next step. (See Figure 76.)

Step Two: Seek and find an area of tenderness directly on top of your head at midline. Sometimes this Oriental acupuncture point is so tender that you can't even touch it with a comb. To this point, apply rotary pressure with the fingertips of either hand. Now put three fingers down in a line extending from this point back and down toward the hollow at the base of your skull. Place your thumb into the hollow. Maintaining this grasp, make the scalp move forward and back on the skull.

Step Three: Now make complete thumb pressure into the hollow. It will be very tender to touch. Just behind the skull plate at this point is the medulla oblongata, and it is in direct communication

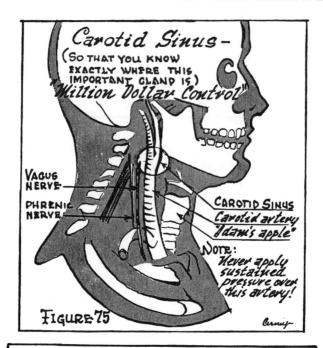

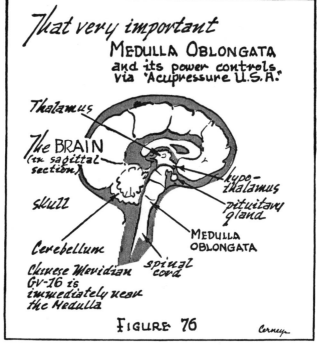

via nerve structure to the area you are compressing. By using this technique, these three steps, you begin to normalize low blood pressure. By this method, the weaknesses of the heart are repaired. By this method, cranial anemia disappears. The mind becomes clear, alert, no longer does that dizzy feeling persist. Your eyes will bother you less and less, and as all of these signs and symptoms disappear, so does low blood pressure. Through the magic of *Acupressure, U.S.A.*, and the complex magnificence of the human body and brain, do you create the miracles of health you desire. (See Figure 77.)

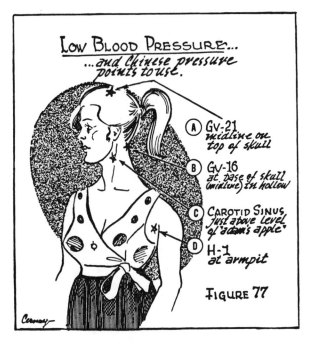

FIGURE 77

HIGH BLOOD PRESSURE

One of the most marvelous procedures available to mankind—for the lowering of high blood pressure—is the use of Oriental acupuncture points without—or with—needles. I use it on myself, but let me tell you the story of Dawson who appeared to have "dropped dead" in my office waiting room.

Dawson had stopped at my office to pick up an insurance payment that had come in for his daughter's x-rays. As he stood there talking to my Girl Friday, he simply keeled over. I applied emergency care on his carotid sinuses and the tips of the little fingers. He came to.

His face was a mask of astonishment as his hands sought his head. He looked up at me and said, "It's gone! That crazy pressure in my head is gone!" That's when I learned Mr. Dawson was a high blood pressure case, that x-rays of his heart had revealed calcified coronary arteries and thick, calcified plaques on the aortic arch. That's when I learned that his heart was failing and the surgeon deemed it necessary for open heart surgery. Blood pressure 260 over 140 . . . the kind doctors hate to see walk into their office because they already belong to the walking dead . . . and Dawson walked into mine.

I called a taxicab and then called his physician. A short time later, the doctor called me back. He was apparently bewildered by the change in Dawson. "What did you do?" he wanted to know, so I described the technique just as I'm describing it here for you. For mild cases of high blood pressure, it is a splendid home procedure to use. For those with chronically high blood pressure, it should be used *only* in an emergency, and the family physician called at once!

ACUPRESSURE, U.S.A. TECHNIQUE
FOR
CONTROLLING HIGH BLOOD PRESSURE

Technique:

Step One: Fingertip pressure on the carotid sinus. Hold for a slow five count. Breathe deeply. Press once more. Let your breath out. Repeat the process at least three times. Do it on both sides of your neck. It may be done left and right simultaneously.

Step Two: Locate bony ridge at base of skull. This ridge runs from ear to ear. Run your fingertips across it. Note the painful areas in the overlying scalp. Apply pressure on each. Repeat at least three times, with increasing amounts of pressure. (Never be rough.)

Step Three: Solar plexus pressure. Place the fingertips of both hands into your solar plexus area. Expel all air from your lungs. Apply pressure. Hold for a slow five count and release. Repeat three times.

Step Four: Excite Pericardial meridian. Grasp the tip of your third finger, squeeze, pull. Repeat alternately five times on each hand. End your *Acupressure, U.S.A.* therapy with—

Step Five: Pressure on the medulla oblongata area at base of skull. Compress, rub, until the tenderness is gone in the scalp and underlying tissues. As the tenderness dissipates, it's proof positive that *Acupressure, U.S.A.* is doing its job inside!

I have taught this procedure to many patients, and as an emergency technique it has already saved a number of lives. Learn the technique! Use it! The life you save may one day be your very own, and you'll owe it all to my Americanized approach to the mysteries that have long been kept hidden in the Orient.

NOTE: *For additional beneficial influences in curbing high blood pressure, use the following* Schedule of Action.

A B C SCHEDULE OF ACTION

A	B	C	D	E
B-54	K-1	Tw-5	Liv-13	P-9

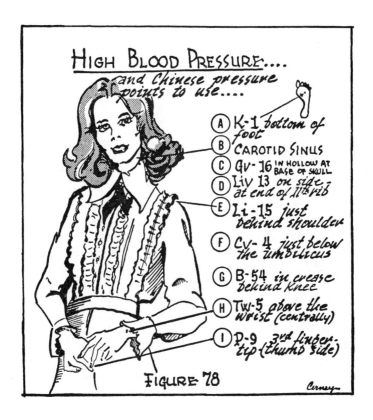

FIGURE 78

"CRICK" IN THE NECK

Cold drafts, air conditioning, sleeping with the head cocked at an angle, direct trauma (blow) to the neck or shoulder muscles, may cause a "crick" in the neck. *Heat and massage should not be used for this problem!* Heat adds more congestion to a part already on fire. Manual manipulation of the muscles during this period also contributes to additional muscle spasm. Then what's the answer? It lies in *Acupressure, U.S.A.* followed by local ice therapy.

Contact the points of spasm. Relax them through pressure. Seek and locate them. Place your thumb into the area. Hold for a three count. Release. Repeat three times, and then begin small rotary pressures until you feel the spasm disappear under your fingertip. Be gentle, *do not pull or push these tissues* at any time. Treat yourself the moment you feel the problem coming on . . . if you are aware of it at all. Follow with a coldpack or ice rub on the points of pain.

A B C SCHEDULE OF ACTION

A	B	C	D	E
Si-15	Tw-15	GB-21	B-10	Gv-16

GOITER

Traditional Chinese doctors felt that when there was a large, hard swelling at the front base of the neck—a swelling that neither moved nor hurt when touched—it was due to *Ch'i* being obstructed, that the blood inside was congealed. Today's physician sees this growth as an enlarged thyroid gland and thinks immediately of iodine substances and inadequate hormone balance.

The simple colloid goiter is due to iodine deficiency and is observed most often in the Great Lakes area, the northwest United States, and the Mississippi valley. Usually such a tumor is unsightly and without symptoms. Sometimes there are complications. Mildred had such a complication. She came here from England where they called this problem "Derbyshire Neck."

Usually a thyroid tumor begins with some flaw in the nervous system. It may start with worry and fright. It may begin with an infection, or it may even be congenital. Mary R.—when she came to my office—presented not only a bulging at the base of her throat, but

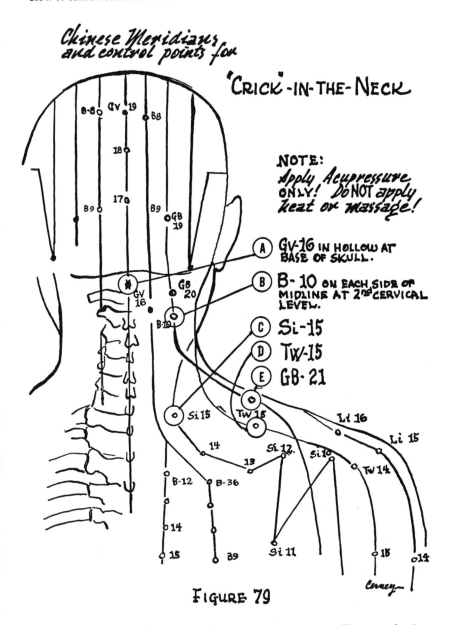

Chinese Meridians and control points for "CRICK"-IN-THE-NECK

NOTE: Apply Acupressure ONLY! Do NOT apply heat or massage!

A) GV-16 IN HOLLOW AT BASE OF SKULL.

B) B-10 ON EACH SIDE OF MIDLINE AT 2ND CERVICAL LEVEL.

C) Si-15

D) Tw-15

E) GB-21

FIGURE 79

also her eyeballs bulged. Her fingers were tremorous. The muscles in her hands and arms twitched. She'd been vomiting and had diarrhea. Her heart beat was very fast. She was anemic, and laboratory tests revealed a high basal metabolism, as well as sugar in the urine. From all indications, Mary had what is called an exophthalmic goiter. She was one of those people who refused to have surgery, so *Acupressure, U.S.A.* was begun.

A B C SCHEDULE OF ACTION

A	B	C	D	E
Gv-20 22 38	B-1 2	S-2 11	H-7	T-10

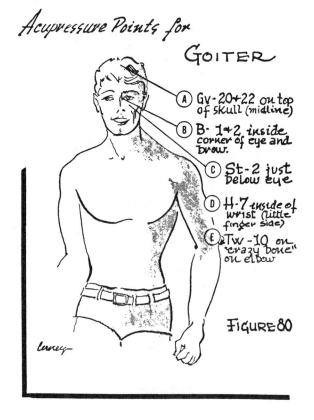

Acupressure Points for

GOITER

Ⓐ Gv-20+22 on top of skull (midline)

Ⓑ B-1+2 inside corner of eye and brow.

Ⓒ St-2 just below eye

Ⓓ H-7 inside of wrist (little finger side)

Ⓔ Tw-10 on "crazy bone" on elbow

FiGURE 80

Supplementary Procedures

1. *Dietary controls.*

   a. Avoid all soybean products and cabbage. Each contains

cyanate which helps produce goiters. Avoid all such drugs that contain this same product.

    b. Use iodized salt at all times (unless your physician instructs otherwise).

    c. Sea kelp may be be added to your diet. It too contains iodine.

    2. *Further acupuncture without needles. (See Figure 81.)*

SUPPLEMENTAL
A B C SCHEDULE OF ACTION

A	B	C	D
St-9 & 27 Carotid -sinus pressure	Cv-22	Gv-15	GB-12

(To locate supplemental "points" also consult other illustrations)

    3. *"Z" zone therapy for thyroid problems.*

Although the Orientals indicate only one acupuncture point (Kidney 1) on the bottom of the foot, the foot is actually replete with important reflex areas. One very important one is that of the thyroid, and in the Americanization of Chinese acupuncture, I prefer to call these plantar reflexes "Z" zones. Each of these "Z" zones is directly related to organs, as well as to the autonomic system . . . as are acupuncture points and meridians. You would do well to take advantage of your own natural resources . . . use the "Z" zones in your hands and feet! Use them to stimulate powerhouses of energy within you. See Figure 23. Check the location of the thyroid "Z" zone and the location of the reflex zones for the pituitary, the pineal, the ovary, the teste, the adrenal, and the parathyroid glands because they structure your well-being.

    Your thyroid "Z" zone is located under the head of the first metatarsal of each foot. On pressure, the "Z" zone will elicit a sharp pain. Use a rotary motion on it with your thumb until the pain is gone. As the pain lessens, the reflex to the thyroid gland—the "race horse of the body"—is being stimulated.

    You are simply not rubbing a sore spot on your foot! Each "Z" zone and the magic of thyroxin flows into the bloodstream. These power activators are at your beck-and-call. You have only to press the "Z" zones and these activators go to work to reduce the collections of waste in your body. They burn up trash. They

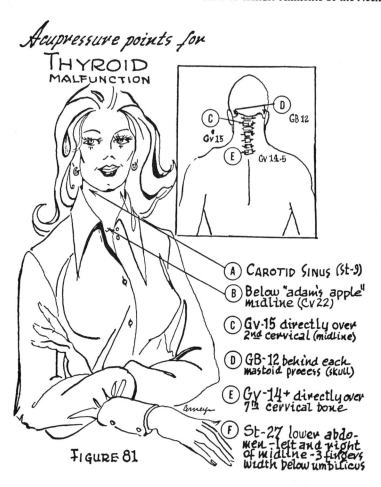

Acupressure points for
THYROID
MALFUNCTION

C — Gv 15
D — GB 12
E — Gv 14-5

(A) CAROTID SINUS (St-9)

(B) Below "adam's apple" midline (Cv 22)

(C) Gv-15 directly over 2nd cervical (midline)

(D) GB-12 behind each mastoid process (skull)

(E) Gv-14+ directly over 7th cervical bone

(F) St-27 lower abdomen—left and right of midline—3 fingers width below umbilicus

FIGURE 81

innervate the other glands and say, "Boys, let's go to work!" But if you don't use these activators—if the thyroid gland in your neck is permitted to fall asleep—that's when you get chronically tired, bored, listless, that's when you keep looking for a place to lie down. Keep in mind that thyroxin is liquid magic. It steps you up for action. It makes you more alert. In this little gland at the front base of your neck, is encapsulated fuel, never ending energy, a quick way to get that added lift when you need it most! The button to do it—your "Z" zone—is in your foot!

LARYNGITIS

Laryngitis may be acute or chronic, and usually results after exposure to cold or wet. It may come from breathing in dust or chemical vapors. Nose or throat infections may trigger it. Measles or whooping cough may start it going. Then there's nerve pressure in the bones of the neck that can do the same thing. Maudie B. was such a case. She'd had laryngitis for years. Off-again, on-again, her larynx was chronically inflamed. She'd get hoarse and lose her speech and her ability to swallow. When all this happened, it interfered with her career. By another more exotic name, you know Maudie as a popular singer, a beautiful gal with personality-plus. But every time she got exposed to manual effort, emotions, or dampness, the laryngitis came on with a bang. Sometimes fumes and dust brought it on. Sometimes shooting for a high note out of her normal vocal range started it going, and all such factors were murder to her hotel and nightclub engagements.

Maudie tried everything. On prescription she took iodides internally. She stopped smoking and laid off alcohol. She had medicated sprays and inhalation therapy. She was checked for possible infections that might be extending to her nose and throat. Galvanocautery was used on her tonsils, and then a specialist suggested gastrostomy and resection of the superior laryngeal nerve. He wouldn't guarantee that she would sing again.

That's when I saw Maudie. She told me about the constant sensation of tickling that she had in her throat, the feeling of rawness, and the constant urge to clear her throat. Sometimes her throat felt "full" and she had difficulty swallowing. Examination and history pointed at chronic laryngitis. X-ray film of her cervical bones revealed something else. Two vertebrae were subluxated from their normal position. Maudie remembered falling off the stage in Los Vegas during a rehearsal and that's when it all began.

The following ABC Schedule of Action is the method used on Maudie after the bones were set back into place. Within a week, Maudie's symptoms were gone. She's back in show business once more. She maintains the schedule I laid down for her. Her health as well as her career depend on the preventive measures she is using. Following is the action I recommended:

A B C SCHEDULE OF ACTION

A	B	C	D	E
Cv-23 22	Gv-5 14	Li-1	St-4	L-1

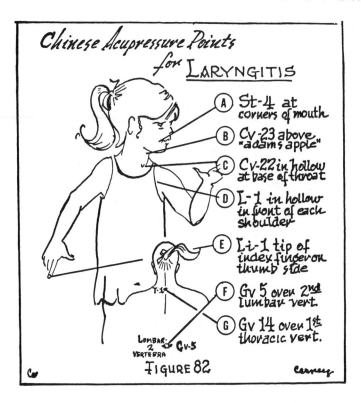

Chinese Acupressure Points for LARYNGITIS

A) St-4 at corners of mouth

B) Cv-23 above "adam's apple"

C) Cv-22 in hollow at base of throat

D) L-1 in hollow in front of each shoulder

E) Li-1 tip of index finger on thumb side

F) Gv 5 over 2nd lumbar vert.

G) Gv 14 over 1st thoracic vert.

FIGURE 82

Supplemental Procedures

1. *Physical therapy.*
    a. *Relieve tension* by massaging neck and back muscles. Also massage the muscles of the upper chest.
    b. *Compress applications:* place a *cold* compress on the back of the neck at the base of the skull and a *hot* compress on the front of the neck.
    c. *Salt water enemas* (1 tablespoonful per quart of water) if bowels are inactive.
2. *Dietary control.*
    a. *Liquid or soft diet* until throat is relieved.
3. *Complete rest.*
    a. Give mind, body, and voice a rest.
4. *Habit controls.*
    a. *Eliminate smoking,* alcoholic beverages, and excesses in everything.

PHARYNGITIS

Pharyngitis is inflammation of the pharynx usually associated with an inflamed and runny nose, with the voice quite often being involved.

Whether this condition is from bacteria or chemicals, Nature responds by bringing in shock troops and often overdoes it. To help Nature regulate itself—and neutralize the inflamed pharynx—here's the suggested acupuncture procedure—without needles—to use.

A B C SCHEDULE OF ACTION

A	B	C	D	E	F
Li-6 9	St-5 6 9	Tw-9 15 16	B-17	GB-20 34	L-6 8

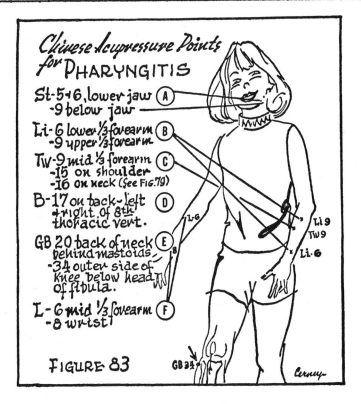

Chinese Acupressure Points
for PHARYNGITIS

St-5 + 6, lower jaw Ⓐ
  -9 below jaw

Li-6 lower ⅓ forearm Ⓑ
  -9 upper ⅓ forearm

Tw-9 mid ⅓ forearm Ⓒ
  -15 on shoulder
  -16 on neck (see Fig.79)

B-17 on back - left Ⓓ
  + right of 8th
  thoracic vert.

GB 20 back of neck Ⓔ
  behind mastoids,
  -34 outer side of
  knee below head
  of fibula.

L-6 mid ⅓ forearm Ⓕ
  -8 wrist

FIGURE 83

Li 9
Tw 9
Li-6
L-6
GB 34

Cerney

**Supplementary
Procedures**

   1. *Physical therapy*
      a. Coldpacks on the *back* of the neck. Hotpacks on the front.
   2. *Dietary controls.*
      a. Add vitamin supplements to your diet (Vitamins A, D, and C).
      b. Soft foods (soup).
      c. No coffee, tea, cola drinks, or milk. You *can* have ginger ale. Avoid frozen and canned fruit juices. They are full of preservatives.
   3. *Avoid all aggravators.*
      a. Avoid chemical, thermal, or other aggravations that precipitate your problem.

SWOLLEN THROAT

When I first saw nine-year-old Nancy, her poor little throat was wrapped in flannel, and some wondrously powerful salve was filling the room with a strange odor reminiscent of bear grease. This cute little kid was having chills, fever, and a headache. She said tearfully, "I feel awful." Her body ached. Her throat hurt when she swallowed, and even the lymph nodes in her neck were protesting. The more she coughed, the stiffer her neck became, and her mother whispered, "Is she getting polio?" Luckily, the course of acute tonsillitis is self-limited, but more serious complications *can* result. To alleviate this possibility, and to bring local relief for swollen throat, here are the *Acupressure, U.S.A.* points to use.

A B C SCHEDULE OF ACTION

A	B	C	D	E	F	G	H
GB-38 40	St-6 40	Si-17 18	Li-1 4	L-3 11	Cv-22	K-1 5	Tw-10

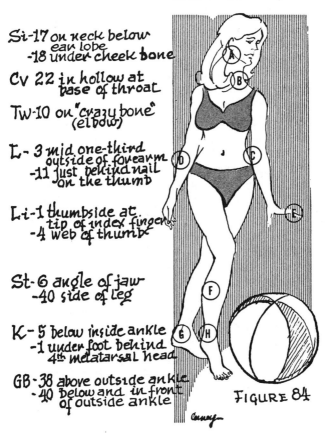

Chinese Acupressure Points
for
SWOLLEN THROAT
(*Acute Tonsilitis*)

Si-17 on neck below
      ear lobe
   -18 under cheek bone

Cv 22 in hollow at
       base of throat

Tw-10 on "crazy bone"
         (elbow)

L- 3 mid one-third
      outside of forearm
   -11 just behind nail
      on the thumb

Li-1 thumbside at
      tip of index finger
   -4 web of thumb

St-6 angle of jaw
   -40 side of leg

K- 5 below inside ankle
   -1 under foot behind
      4th metatarsal head

GB-38 above outside ankle
    -40 below and in front
        of outside ankle

FIGURE 84

Supplemental Procedures

1. *Physical therapy.*
    a. Coldpacks on throat twice daily. *Technique:* Fold a turkish towel lengthwise into a width that will fit your throat. Saturate in cold water. Encircle the throat as many times as the length of the toweling will go. As soon as it warms inside (put

your finger in between toweling and neck), remove and saturate with cold water once more. Repeat as often as desired.
2. *Dietary controls.*
   a. Soft foods only (soups).
   b. Dietary supplements: Vitamins A, D, C.
   c. *No milk!*

TONSILLITIS

Lymph glands protect us against infection. When you get an infection in your foot, the lymph glands in your groin swell to handle the infective problem. No sensible surgeon surgically removes them because the glands have enlarged to do their job. This also applies to tonsillar lymph nodes in the neck.

Tonsils should never be removed unless they are specifically diseased beyond healing. In acute tonsillitis, the onset quite often is sudden. There may be chills. Fever may go to 106°F and malaise, headaches, and body aches accompany it. As these glands swell, the neck tends to stiffen. The tonsils enlarge, get red, exudate collects in the crypts. As in quinsy they may even abscess, and severe pains ensue. In chronic tonsillitis, the adenoid tissue may also be involved.

A complete physical examination and lab workup on Marybeth revealed nothing but a skinny kid with swollen tonsils. There were a few exceptions—certain acupuncture points were extremely tender. Marybeth jumped when they were touched. Her eyes got big. "What in the world is that?" her mother wanted to know, and I told her about acupuncture and how the Chinese doctors insert needles in such areas to get a return of health.

"Are you going to stick needles in me?" Marybeth wanted to know in wide-eyed fear, and I shook my head no. I explained *Acupressure, U.S.A.* procedures and healed Marybeth. You can do the same for you and yours at home.

A B C SCHEDULE OF ACTION

A	B	C	D	E	F
Cv-22	Si-17	L-6 10	Gv-13	Tw-10	Li-4 20

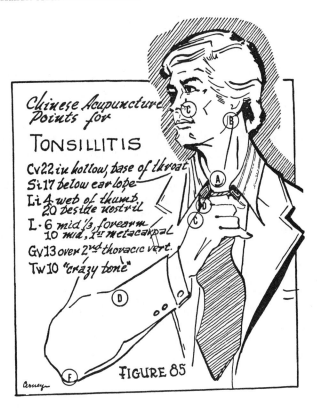

Chinese Acupuncture Points for

TONSILLITIS

Cv 22 in hollow, base of throat
Si 17 below ear lobe
Li 4 web of thumb,
20 beside nostril
L·6 mid ⅓, forearm
10 mid, 1ˢᵗ metacarpal
Gv 13 over 2ⁿᵈ thoracic vert.
Tw 10 "crazy bone"

FIGURE 85

Supplementary Procedures

1. *Physical therapy.*
   a. *Massage.* Relax all muscles of the throat gently. Relax those of the back and chest.
   b. *Coldpacks.* Use as prescribed for "swollen throat." This method is wonderful for relaxation and inducing sleep.
   c. *Salt water irrigation* of bowel (1 tablespoon of salt per quart of water). Also sniff salt water up into the nose.
2. *Dietary controls.*
   a. Maintain a light or liquid diet.
   b. Drink ginger ale. *No* milk!

WHIPLASH INJURY

How Neck Injury Sets Up a Host of Crazy Symptoms Through the Sympathetic Nervous System

Reflex stimulation of the *Sympathetic Nervous System* by way of a rear-end auto collision can give rise to many signs and symptoms that seem totally unrelated to the neck problem at hand. When neck nerves or cervical roots are compressed or traumatized, a train of secondary effects follow. There may be blurring of vision, dilatation of the pupils of the eye, loss of balance, headaches, swelling and stiffness of the fingers, tendonitis, and capsulitis.

A sudden forceful whipping of the head on the neck stretches not just the ligaments that bind the vertebrae, but the muscles that support and maintain the integrity of the spinal bones. It stretches the nervous system as well. The sympathetic nervous system is especially involved. Symptoms of whiplash may occur immediately. Some signs and symptoms may show up years later, and by this time the person who sustained the accident has already forgotten the incident that has brought on the current problem.

Whiplash Injury, and How to Conquer Destruction That Is Destined to Follow

As a specialist in this field, I have been able to tabulate a long list of problems that follow in the wake of automobile accidents and cervico-myofascitis (whiplash injury).

Jack D. was one of those involved in an 18-car pileup. When I saw Jack, his neck was swollen from head to shoulders. In addition to the usual stiff neck, he had a lot of everything else. Shoulder muscles became spasmodic. With the restricted neck and head motion, came headaches, mental dullness, fatigue, and blackouts. He was disoriented at times. His head, neck, and shoulders "felt heavy." Numbness occurred in his arms, shoulders, hands, feet, and legs.

Like other whiplash victims, he became extremely "nervous." He had a change of personality. There was ringing in his ears. He had a shortness of breath, nausea, and a desire to vomit. He had a low back pain, pain between the shoulder blades, cold hands and feet, and excessive sweating. And that wasn't all. With his growing irritability, came loss of memory. He couldn't remember what happened in the accident. He couldn't concentrate. He was easily depressed and showed anxiety at all times. His heart beat rapidly, and he kept squinting as if fighting the light. He couldn't sleep. He was living through hell, and he went from doctor to doctor looking for relief. Most of them indicated his symptoms were fancied. One of them said he was just goofing-off.

Neuro-surgeons put him through the mill, and after a tenure in the hospital he still had his hurts. After six months of this, he came into my office. Elongated history taking and physical examination all dropped into a pattern—cervico-myofascitis, whiplash injury, and an excellent case for acupuncture. Although needles were used in Jack's case, he was given a diagram of the same acupuncture points to hand-treat at home. In a month's time, he was back at work. No surgery! No further loss of time. Within the week he was sleeping all night, and his pains dropped away one by one. The sympathetic system re-established itself and Jack D.'s pains were gone. Now, just like he regularly services his car, he brings himself in for rehabilitative therapy, and here is the ABC program we follow.

A B C SCHEDULE OF ACTION

A	B	C	D	E	F	G
Cv-22	St 11	Gv-14 16 20 22	GB-20	B-10	Li-4 6	L-5

See Figure 86 for details on above A B C Chart.

TORTICOLLIS

How It Gets you in the Neck Every Time

Torticollis is a stiff neck caused by spasmodic contractions of muscles of the neck, drawing the head to one side with the chin pointing opposite to the side of the contraction.

Sometimes called "wryneck," it is the flexion or drawing of the head toward one shoulder on the side of the contracted muscle ... but not the chin. The head may rotate or extend in an awkward position, and with these muscles in spasm, it is a problem that is hard to treat under any circumstance.

The onset may be slow and insidious. It may come suddenly. The trapezius muscles, the splenius capitus, sternocleidomastoid, and splenius collis muscles start pulling, and the head moves in the direction of the spasm. If it lasts very long, the neck muscles on that side begin to thicken as well as shorten.

The Case of Mrs. "X."

X-ray film of Mrs. X.'s neck revealed that the first cervical vertebra, the one the head sits on, was subluxated out of its normal alignment. Her head was actually off its base, and years of muscle spasm complicated the reduction of this dislocation. So we started with a mild massage program on the neck, shoulders, and chest. The patient was told to use coldpacks on her neck and upper back daily following each massage. This was done every day for two weeks. Muscles began to relax and acupuncture without needles began.

One month later, I sent Mrs. X. back to her local surgeon. He just shook his head and marvelled at the improvement. He told her he was pleased at her progress and wanted to know what had been done to achieve it? She told him. Here's the acupuncture point schedule we followed.

A B C SCHEDULE OF ACTION

A	B	C	D	E	F	G
Gv-14 16	GB-20	L-5	Cv-22	St-11	B-10	Li-4 16

(See Figure 86 for details on above ABC Chart.)

**Supplementary
Procedures**

    1. *Physical therapy.*

       (a) *Massage* neck, shoulder, and chest muscles. Massage them daily.

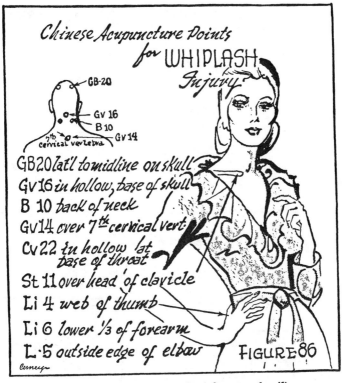

Chinese Acupuncture Points
for WHIPLASH *Injury*

GB-20
Gv 16
B 10
Gv 14
7th cervical vertebra

GB 20 *lat'l to midline on skull*
Gv 16 *in hollow, base of skull*
B 10 *back of neck*
Gv 14 *over 7th cervical vert*
Cv 22 *in hollow 'at base of throat*
St 11 *over head 'of clavicle*
Li 4 *web of thumb*
Li 6 *lower 1/3 of forearm*
L·5 *outside edge of elbow*

FIGURE 86

(See Figure 13 and 14 for arm detail)

(b) *Cold compresses* on the back of the neck and shoulder at least an hour each day.

(c) *Remove the cause.*

(d) *Compression over the medulla oblongata area.* Technique: To tune up the entire autonomic nervous system, for torticollis or whiplash therapy, place the ball of your thumb directly into the hollow at the base of your skull. Seek and find the painful areas in this key midline acupuncture point (Gv-16) and maintain pressure until the pain subsides.

(e) *Follow the occipital ridge.* From ear to ear, at the base of the skull, you will find a ridge. Follow this bony abutment with your fingertips. Note the areas of tenderness and swelling that exist along its entire course. Mark them as vital treatment points. Compress each with your thumb with a massagic, rotary motion. Be gentle but firm. Treat all such "ouch areas" equally. When there is the least suggestion of cervical injury, apply

Acupressure, U.S.A. immediately. There are *no contraindications* to this type of care!

BONUS THERAPIES
FOR ADDITIONAL NECK PROBLEMS

NOTE: *Full-page drawings follow now on the acupuncture pressure point care of:*

1. *Stiff Neck* (Other Than Whiplash).
2. *Pedal Pressure Points—"Z" Zones for Relaxing Neck and Shoulders.*

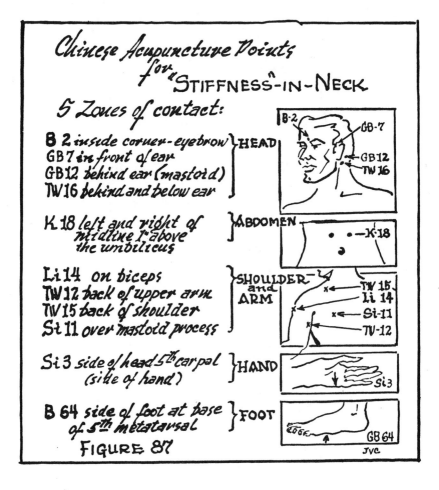

Chinese Acupuncture Points
for "STIFFNESS"-IN-NECK

5 Zones of contact:

B 2 *inside corner-eyebrow* }HEAD
GB 7 *in front of ear*
GB 12 *behind ear (mastoid)*
TW 16 *behind and below ear*

K 18 *left and right of midline 1" above the umbilicus* }ABDOMEN

Li 14 *on biceps* }SHOULDER and ARM
TW 12 *back of upper arm*
TW 15 *back of shoulder*
St 11 *over mastoid process*

Si 3 *side of hand 5th carpal (side of hand)* }HAND

B 64 *side of foot at base of 5th metatarsal* }FOOT

FIGURE 87

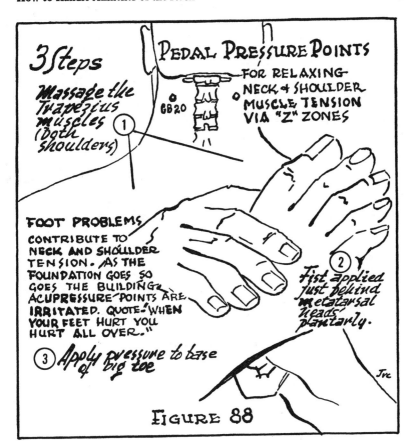

3 Steps

Massage the Trapezius muscles (both shoulders) ①

PEDAL PRESSURE POINTS
FOR RELAXING NECK & SHOULDER MUSCLE TENSION VIA "Z" ZONES

o GB20

FOOT PROBLEMS CONTRIBUTE TO NECK AND SHOULDER TENSION. AS THE FOUNDATION GOES SO GOES THE BUILDING. ACUPRESSURE POINTS ARE IRRITATED. QUOTE "WHEN YOUR FEET HURT YOU HURT ALL OVER."

② Fist applied just behind metatarsal heads plantarly.

③ Apply pressure to base of big toe

Jvc

FIGURE 88

HOW TO HANDLE
AILMENTS OF THE CHEST

6

Following are acupressure techniques for:

> Asthma
> Bronchitis
> Heart Problems
> > Angina Pectoris
> > Bradycardia
> > Pericarditis

Also there are additional therapies for:

Influenza
Chest Muscle Spasm

CHEST PAIN . . . AND
HOW TO IDENTIFY ITS SOURCE

Marilyn M. had a problem. She had a pain. She said, "The pain is in my lungs," not knowing that lung tissue has little or no sensitivity. This made her self-diagnosis somewhat improbable, but it also indicated the fact that sometimes it is difficult to identify the source of a pain if you are not knowledgeable about the intricacies of the human body.

Pain she had, and it was our job to find from whence it came.

There are many causes of pain in the chest. They may be inside the chest cavity, in soft tissue, or in bone (ribs, vertebrae). Or, they may be referred from other body parts. Pain in the chest cavity may be transferred from the pleural sac and be called pleurisy. It may stem from the bronchial tubes or bronchus. Pleuritis may manifest itself under the ribs. In pneumonia, the pain may not be in the lungs but refers itself into the abdomen instead. When the pleura is involved, pain may shoot up into the left shoulder or to a point above the clavicle—and when you use Chinese acupuncture, this must be remembered!

To save a lot of time and explanation, the following illustrations make it precisely plain. It also points up the fact that you shouldn't try to diagnose your own chest problems. When the diagnosis is

CAUSES of CHEST PAIN

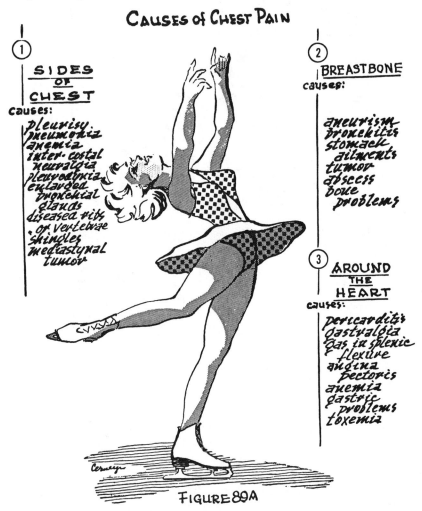

① SIDES OF CHEST
causes:
pleurisy,
pneumonia
anemia
inter-costal
neuralgia
pleurodynia,
enlarged
bronchial
glands
diseased ribs
or vertebrae
shingles
mediastynal
tumor

② BREASTBONE
causes:
aneurism
bronchitis
stomach
ailments
tumor
abscess
bone
problems

③ AROUND THE HEART
causes:
pericarditis
gastralgia
gas in splenic
flexure
angina
pectoris
anemia
gastric
problems
toxemia

FIGURE 89A

already known, you can use *acupuncture—without needles*—to your advantage. Such problems as asthma, bronchitis, and heart problems are dealt with here. See Figures 89A and 89B.

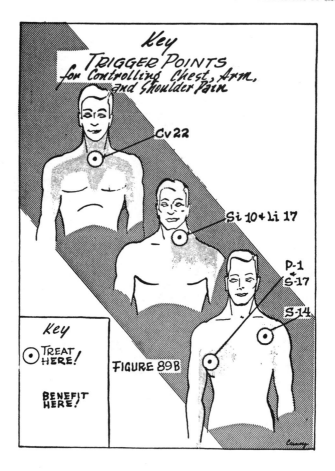

Key
TRIGGER POINTS
for Controlling Chest, Arm, and Shoulder Pain

Cv 22

Si 10 + Li 17

P-1
S-17

S-14

Key
⊙ TREAT HERE!

BENEFIT HERE!

FIGURE 89B

ASTHMA

Asthma may be caused by an allergy or some imflammatory change in the bronchial tree. Allergies may come from hayfever, dusts, foods, and bacteria. Tendencies toward asthma may be inherited. Fatigue and emotions may bring it on. Damp and cold weather are aggravators. I watched it occur with a young mother in her first pregnancy. After the delivery, the asthma was gone. Another young lady we'll call Della said she'd had asthma since childhood and that she would vomit and itch all over during an "attack." Asthma may come on suddenly or it may creep up unnoticed. When Jean R. had it for the first time, she experienced gas in her abdomen, felt chilly, and was depressed. Her chest felt full. Her nose and throat itched. Breathing became more and more difficult, and a feeling of suffocation developed. Coughing ended with expectoration. Significant in Jean's case was the fact that between "attacks," all her signs and symptoms of asthma disappeared completely. The acupressure procedure we used to get her back to health is as follows.

A B C SCHEDULE OF ACTION

A	B	C	D	E	F	G
Gv-12	Li-4 14	Sp-8 9	Liv-2	St-4	Si-4	L-1

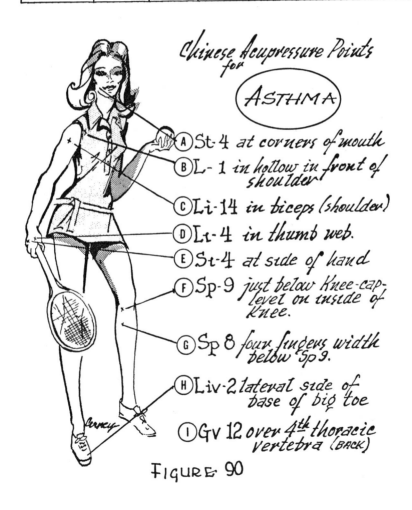

Chinese Acupressure Points
for

(ASTHMA)

(A) St-4 at corners of mouth
(B) L-1 in hollow in front of shoulder
(C) Li-14 in biceps (shoulder)
(D) Li-4 in thumb web.
(E) St-4 at side of hand
(F) Sp-9 just below knee-cap-level on inside of knee.
(G) Sp 8 four fingers width below Sp 9.
(H) Liv-2 lateral side of base of big toe
(I) Gv 12 over 4th thoracic vertebra (BACK)

FIGURE 90

1. *Physical therapy.*
(a) *Heat* applied over thoracic vertebrae when the problem occurs at night. Alternate once per week with a coldpack over the same area. Time: 30 minutes.
(b) *Massage muscles* of back, neck, and chest three times weekly.
(c) *Vibrate all pressure points* or "bumps" that are palpated high on the chest wall.
2. *Dietary control.*
Eat *no heavy meals* at any time. Eat no evening meals at all. Eat no sweets or gas-forming foods.

BRONCHITIS

During the beginning stages of this problem, there is an irritating cough. It's a dry, rough, paroxysmal cough. As the mucous membrane dries out, there is a feeling of discomfort, pain, or fullness in the chest. Breathing may become difficult. Chest pain is the second big symptom. It may be a "tickling" type pain or it may actually become "raw." Stabbing pain may be felt during periods of coughing. Fever may go to 103° F and a headache may occur. The necessity here in treating bronchitis is to produce a skin hyperemia.

How a Factory Worker
Was "Cured"

Bronchitis may be chronic or acute. When factory worker Tom T. had his acute case of bronchitis, he said he felt tired, uncomfortable, and that he breathed with difficulty. He felt slightly sore under his breastbone. Sometimes it felt like something constricting him. Coughing at first was wracking and painful. It was dry. Expectoration came up later as the inflammation cooled off. Tom tried various therapies but his bronchitis continued. It became chronic. In chronic bronchitis, the cough is persistent. He developed a nagging soreness under his breastbone. With exertion he began to have trouble breathing. He had no fever, but he did spit up a lot, and the phlegm was quite foul. Acupuncture and *Acupressure, U.S.A.* were begun. He had immediately good results. Within a month, all residual symptoms were gone. The schedule of action used is as follows:

A B C SCHEDULE OF ACTION

A	B	C	D	E
Gv-12	Cv-21	Sp-16	L-1 8	H-3

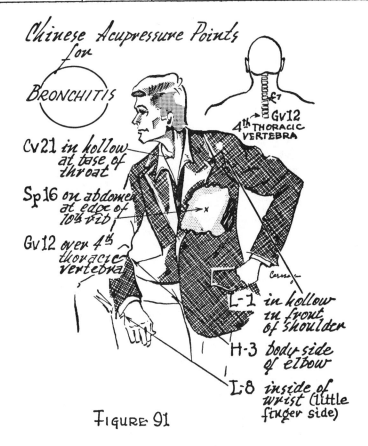

Chinese Acupressure Points for

BRONCHITIS

Cv 21 in hollow at base of throat

Sp 16 on abdomen at edge of 10th rib

Gv 12 over 4th thoracic vertebra

C7

Gv 12 4th THORACIC VERTEBRA

×

L-1 in hollow in front of shoulder

H-3 body side of elbow

L-8 inside of wrist (little finger side)

FIGURE 91

Supplementary Procedures

    1. *Physical therapy.*
        (a) Hot mustard footbath.
        (b) Mild mustard plaster to the chest (re-apply every eight hours).

(c) Massage neck, chest, and back muscles daily.

(d) Warm, moist air to soothe a dry cough. *Do not use medicated steam.* All volatile oils rising from a vaporizer are irritants! This you don't need.

2. *Dietary controls.*

(a) Fluids in abundance (juices).

(b) Light diet (soups).

3. *Other controls.*

(a) Keep bowels and kidneys active.

(b) Stay in bed during acute "attacks," even if there is no fever. Keep windows open.

(c) Avoid all smoke, dust, fumes.

(d) Avoid extremes of hot, cold, moisture.

4. *Bonus procedures.*

(a) Where nose is runny and there is a minor cough and chills, use L-8 as your acupuncture point.

(b) Where there is hard coughing, painful breathing, phlegm, and the chest feels heavy, use L-5, 8, and 9 acupuncture points. If your treatment has been effective, you can go to L-1 to cross-check as to the effectiveness of your therapy. It will be painless if what you have done has worked.

HEART PROBLEMS

Too often, because of our ignorance, we never take advantage of acupuncture points that can restore our health. Where the heart is concerned, this is especially true.

In the early stages of developing acupuncture, the Chinese located 650 or more of these acupuncture points. In personally checking these little trigger points, I found microscopically that these points—located in and just beneath the skin—are not always over the same kinds of tissue. Some acupuncture points may be palpated as actual hollows. Some are located over muscle contractions, some over nerve bundles, some over bifurcations of venous vessels, some over the valves of veins—and the latter is the most significant in the cardiac patient.

In examining patients with cardiac problems, I find they have areas of exquisite tenderness over the left breast, in the left armpit, and down the left arm to the wrist.

In experimenting on myself—as an angina pectoris victim—I located these trigger points on my chest and arm. Further investigation revealed that these same "points" overlayed vein valves. The valves were apparently closed, because as soon as they were vibrated with acupressure, the anginal pain stopped. After checking your chest for these key areas, probe between your ribs. Vibrate each little "bump" you find. Do it gently. Now follow up the neck along the jugular vein. This too—if you are having heart problems—will exhibit areas of tenderness.

How Rosemary D. Was "Cured"

Rosemary D. had constant attacks of what one doctor called "asthma," and another said it was a cardiac attack. For 40 years this dear old lady had gone faithfully to doctors with her "asthma," and it was her cross to bear. The attacks were usually abrupt. When they came, she had a sense of tightness in her chest, and she wheezed like a sick race horse. Sometimes this lasted for days. Then she'd start coughing and up would come foul, thick sputum. When this came up, she felt relieved. A stethoscopic check of her heart and lungs dialed in raucous, sibilant, and sonorous sounds that made nothing identifiable.

Her chest was a mass of little bumps beneath the skin. The little bumps went deep into the underlying tissue. They disappeared under gentle acupressure vibration. More amazing was the fact that when they disappeared, so did the "asthma."

With this information under my clinic coat, I checked under her left foot for that all-important "Z" zone in the heart area. It was exquisitely tender. I rubbed the pain out of this spot and followed this by compressing the second and third toes together.

The dear lady looked down at me. She grinned and said, "I don't know what you're doing down there, but I'm breathing easier now."

She was instructed on how to use acupuncture pressure points on herself and how to include her little venous bumps in the self-examination. Since that original examination and treatment, she hasn't had one return of her complaint. Her "asthma" was gone! Hard to believe? Yes indeed, but what proved effective for her has proven effective with every patient since with the same problem.

Angina Pectoris

Angina pectoris is an oppressive pain about the heart and under the sternum, with agony radiating to the shoulder and left arm.

Cause: some involvement of the coronary arteries, the heart wall, or the aortic heart valves.

Any person experiencing this pain may also experience anxiety, fear, and even feel that death is near. His face may get livid. It may also get ashen. His face sweats. His pulse is fast. Blood pressure goes up. Pain may last a few seconds, or for what seems to be endless time. To cope with it immediately, vibrate out the little sore areas in your chest and arm. Then apply pressure to the following key acupressure points:

A B C SCHEDULE OF ACTION

A	B	C	D	E
St-15	B-12 21	Cv-14	GB-42	K-1

Supplementary Procedures   (See Figure 92)

1. *Physical therapy.*

(a) *Muscle massage.* Get the muscles of the upper back and neck relaxed by a buddy. Note where particular spots are tender. Have him mark them. These are acupuncture points. Place thumb pressure on them. Hold. Release. Vibrate the area with acupressure until the local tension is dissipated. The organ with which it is associated will be back to working at par.

(b) *Exercise.* Place the fingertips of your right hand into the hollow behind your *left* clavicle. Lock down. Now raise your left arm sideways. Repeat five times despite the tenderness. Now switch to the other side with the opposite hand. Elevate the right arm and lower it five times.

2. *Dietary controls.*

(a) *Vitamin E* added to the diet. This product should be from natural sources only!

(b) *Fast* at least one day each week. If you find it impossible to go without food, eat grapes. Eat as many grapes as you desire.

How to Tune Up Your Heart
for Healthful Action Each Day

Anyone with angina pectoris or any other involvement of the

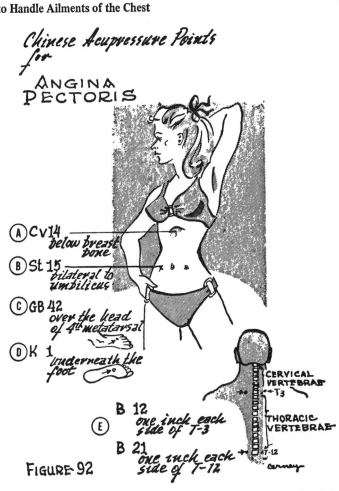

Chinese Acupressure Points for

ANGINA PECTORIS

(A) Cv14 *below breast bone*

(B) St 15 *bilateral to umbilicus*

(C) GB 42 *over the head of 4th metatarsal*

(D) K 1 *underneath the foot*

(E) B 12 *one inch each side of T-3*

B 21 *one inch each side of T-12*

CERVICAL VERTEBRAE
←T3

THORACIC VERTEBRAE
←T-12

Conway

FIGURE 92

heart should be interested in a method of conditioning both heart and body for the hard usage that each gets each day.

Modern living has contributed to tremendous pressures on the human heart, and anything that can be done to condition and maintain its strength and capability should be used.

This same modern living, on the other hand, contributes to sets of conditions that create sites of pains that are false cardiac-like pains and may be most misleading. There may be palpitations, discomfort in the heart area, and "loss of wind," and all may be symptoms that appear to be the real thing. In turn, all may be due to factors causing an imbalance in the autonomic nervous system, and for this there has to be an answer.

Acupressure, U.S.A. which deals directly with the autonomic nervous system, is a direct answer, not just to tuning your heart up for action but for counteracting stress. It is an answer to neurotic behavior that may damage the heart as well as destroy abnormal metabolism and the body's intricate systems.

Acupressure, U.S.A., as a regulating agent with dynamic powers, can even control such a powerhouse as the hypothalamus gland in the midbrain. By regulating the hypothalamus, *Acupressure, U.S.A.* usually makes "symptoms go away." Palpitations of the heart and other erratic cardiac misbehavior disappear. Breathing normalizes. Discomforts in the chest usually go away.

But whether the heart pains are real, or whether they have been induced by neurotic thinking, *Acupressure, U.S.A.* is the treatment of choice to regulate them. In the following procedure, taken from therapies of the Orient, you have a secret weapon for preserving your health and perpetuating your life. You have a way of coping with modern life and staying ahead of the game, keeping active, being a front-line runner, having energy and go-power to get your job done, whether you are a big corporate executive or a housewife.

How to Take Less Than Ten Minutes a Day to Tune Yourself Up for Action

Technique

1. *Stimulate the Heart Meridian.* Grasp the tip of the little finger and whirl it around and around. Pause. Pull on the little finger, bend it in toward the palm. Then start whirling it again. Five seconds does it. Now squeeze the tip of the third finger on each hand. Hold. Squeeze three times.

2. *Pressurize the "Z" Zone in Your Left Foot.* A powerful reflex zone is present just behind the fourth metatarsal head on the bottom of your left foot! Use it to tune yourself up to top performance. Do it each morning as you get out of bed. Do it regularly!

3. *Remove Acupuncture Point Pain in the Chest Wall.* Locate all tension areas in the left chest. There may be a few on the right. Nodule-like "bumps" will be in the pectoralis muscle. Usually they are above the nipple line. Compress them till they disappear. Use the same seek-and-find method to locate these same "nodules" in the armpit and down the inside of the left arm. Check the right arm as well. Apply pressure on the *Heart meridian* at intervals all the way down to the little finger.

4. *Use the Solar Plexus Tension-Release System.* Place the fingertips of each hand into the solar plexus area. Press for the three count. Release. Take deep breath. Release. Apply pressure once more. Repeat five times.

5. *Spinal Nerve Stimulation Procedure.* Stand with your back to the edge of a doorframe. Lean back into it. Locate the sore spots between your scapula and spinal column on the side first. Press back into it. In so doing, you are stimulating the spinal nerve to the heart. You are mechanically causing a message to be sent to the brain, which in turn tells the heart to go to work with renewed vigor.

6. *Use Your Governing Vessel Meridian Efficiently.* At the top of your skull, you will locate a sore spot. There may be more down the centerline toward your spine. Pressurize all of these key "buttons," because each generates energy to improve your day.

7. *The Final Master-Touch Is in the Medulla Oblongata Area!* For that final autonomic power stimulus, turn to the big master switch. Acupuncture point Gv-16 (*Governing Vessel meridian*) is the key button to press. This master tune-up point is in the hollow at the base of the skull. Apply your thumbs or third fingers into this hollow. Massage the area until the pain is gone. Then run the same fingers down either side of the spinal column and ease away the muscle tension.

You've invested less than ten minutes to insure yourself against the pressures of modern living and its ravages upon the human heart. Use this morning tune-up with your Pre-Breakfast Routine. Combine the two in a total routine, and they can change the course of your life.

Bradycardia (Slow Heart Beat)

The very slow beat of the heart—less than 50 beats per minute—elevates only when the individual becomes overheated, emotional, or overly active. In sinus bradycardia, a person with such a problem may have frequent fainting spells and vertigo. The problem may occur even during slumber. It may be precipitated by an infection. It may even happen during an "attack" of jaundice. In other words, anything that brings pressure to bear on the heart will slow it down. To treat it with *Acupressure, U.S.A.*, use the same procedure as for angina pectoris.

Supplementary
Procedures

1. *Lie down if faintness is experienced.*

2. *Never wear tight clothing or tight collars.*

3. *Apply hot applications* (dry or wet) over the spinal column from the second to the sixth thoracic vertebra. (One hour per day.) When the heart begins to speed its pace, use the treatment only three times a week and gradually wean away from therapy in just this manner.

Pericarditis

Pericarditis is inflammation of the pericardium (sac) that surrounds the heart.

Quite often this condition happens to folks who have had rheumatic fever or some involvement of the kidneys. Infection is essentially the major cause (pneumonia, tonsillitis, scarlet fever, tuberculosis, uremia, etc.).

Pain, at the onset, is usually experienced the way Bobby Joe C. experienced it. Bobby Joe was a railroad car inspector. He was constantly on the go and looked forward to retirement, which was just a few years away. What was bothering him was that he was afraid the Company doctor would learn about his chest pain and that he'd get fired, and not get retirement funds to which he was entitled after 30 years with the Line.

His chest pain began at the very tip of the sternum (breast-bone). Sometimes he felt it in his abdomen. It was an anginal-type pain that was sharp and stabbing, and coughing made it worse. Deep breathing aggravated it. When he got in and out of those railroad cars, the exertion started it going and he fell back in pain. A day at the Yard was agony, and every morning it kept getting harder and harder to face the day. The chest pain got so terrible that Bobby Joe finally had to seek professional care. Acupuncture and acupressure was used effectively. He made it! He's in retirement now. Felt so good, he went and got a younger wife.

A B C SCHEDULE OF ACTION

A	B	C	D
H-1 7 8	Cv-14	K-1	B-1

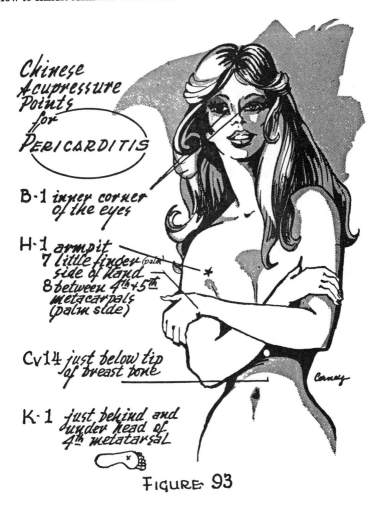

Chinese
Acupressure
Points
for
PERICARDITIS

B·1 inner corner
of the eyes

H·1 armpit
7 little finger (palm)
side of hand
8 between 4th+5th
metacarpals
(palm side)

Cv14 just below tip
of breast bone

K·1 just behind and
under head of
4th metatarsal

FIGURE 93

**Supplemental
Procedures**

1. *Physical therapy.*

(a) Complete rest for the heart, body, and mind.

(b) Icebag over the sixth cervical to the sixth thoracic vertebra. Twice daily—30 minutes each day.

(c) *Icebag over the heart* (one hour each day). NOTE: *Remove icebag every 15 minutes. Rub the skin until glowing. Replace icepack.*

(d) *Apply hotpack to the left side of the neck* (vagus nerve)—30 minutes per treatment—three times weekly.

(e) Massage deeply into the abdomen each day. Keep upper back and neck massaged as well.

2. *Keep away from all excitement.*

3. *Keep kidneys, bowels, and liver active.*

4. *DON'Ts to develop:*

(a) *Don't* get involved. Walk away from trouble!

(b) *Don't* eat heavily. Eat lightly of soups and liquids.

(c) *Don't* participate in smoking, alcohol, or too active exercise.

BONUS THERAPIES

NOTE: An illustration follows on *Acupressure, U.S.A. Techniques for influenza* (where lungs are involved).

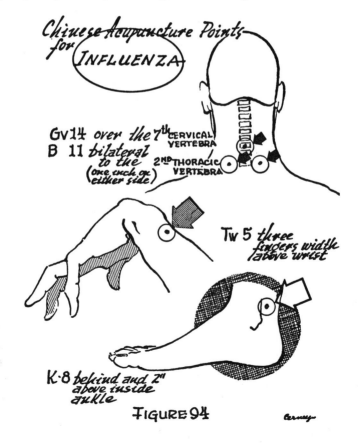

Chinese Acupuncture Points for INFLUENZA

Gv14 over the 7th CERVICAL VERTEBRA
B 11 bilateral to the 2ND THORACIC VERTEBRA (one inch on either side)

Tw 5 three fingers width above wrist

K·8 behind and 2" above inside ankle

FIGURE 94

UPPER EXTREMITIES

THE SHOULDER

The shoulder is a shallow ball-and-socket joint that is highly susceptible to injury. It remains intact only so long as its ligaments, joint capsule, tendons, nerve and blood supply, lymph system, bone position, muscle power, and acupuncture meridians remain intact. Violate one or more of the agents and the shoulder is impaired. Pain in one form or another begins.

Illustrations following will show you "what to do and where" when shoulder problems are involved.

There are certain shoulder pains associated primarily with fatigue and neurasthenia. Some people have very relaxed joints and no problems. Skinny people with loose muscles usually have a relaxed joint. Heavy, muscular people tend to be stiff and have restricted shoulder movement. When a joint is chronically involved, the muscles that control it tend to atrophy and/or shrink. Atrophy of the big deltoid muscle is characteristic of a disused or frozen shoulder.

At all times remember that movements—not muscles—are the functional units in the central nervous system, as well as the Chinese acupuncture meridian system—and when the shoulder and upper extremity are involved by some pain, direct or indirect injury, *all* soft tissues, as well as bone, are involved! *No injury is ever local. No pain or hurt is ever confined to any one given spot or area!* It's the old story—when your feet hurt, you hurt all over! When you've got a bad headache, you're even "sick to your stomach."

Since the following illustrations are self-explanatory, no comments will accompany them. Use regular *Acupressure, U.S.A.* pressure techniques as physical therapy. Physical therapeutics with acupuncture pressure points is essentially the same for the upper extremity. Viz: (a) *hotpacks*, (b) *massage* deep but gently and never over the site of the injury or pain, (c) *progressive exercises* to be used until the arm—executing a complete rotation at the shoulder—makes the excursion without discomfort or stress.

Two types of pain control follow: (1) *Trigger-Point Control* or regional pain. The following illustrations (Figures 95-97B) pinpoint exactly where these triggers are. Combine trigger-point therapy with *Acupressure* procedures. (2) *Acupressure, U.S.A.* points in Brief-at-a-Glance ABC's of Action. Seek your symptom on the chart. Check the accompanying illustration. Find the pressure point on yourself. Probe. Mark. Apply proper therapy.

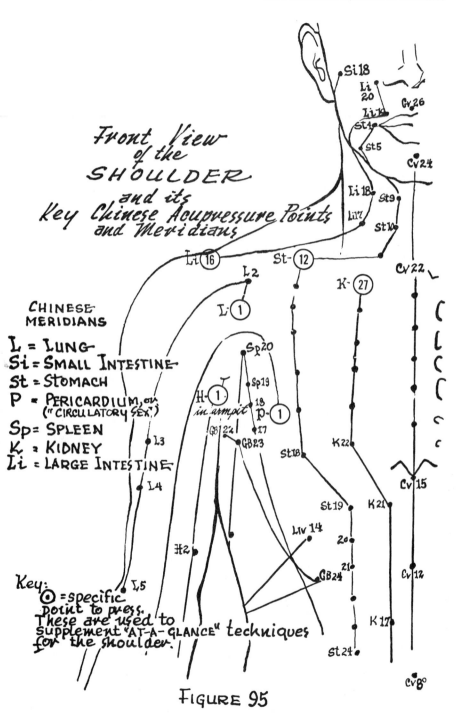

FIGURE 95

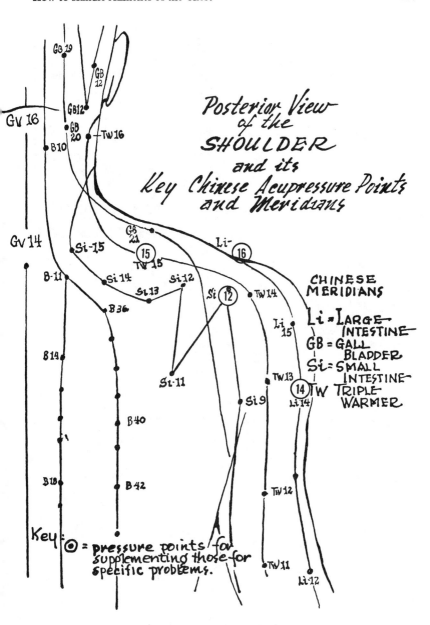

Posterior View
of the
SHOULDER
and its
Key Chinese Acupressure Points
and Meridians

CHINESE
MERIDIANS

Li = LARGE
INTESTINE
GB = GALL
BLADDER
Si = SMALL
INTESTINE
TW TRIPLE
WARMER

Key: ◉ = pressure points for
supplementing those for
specific problems.

FIGURE 96

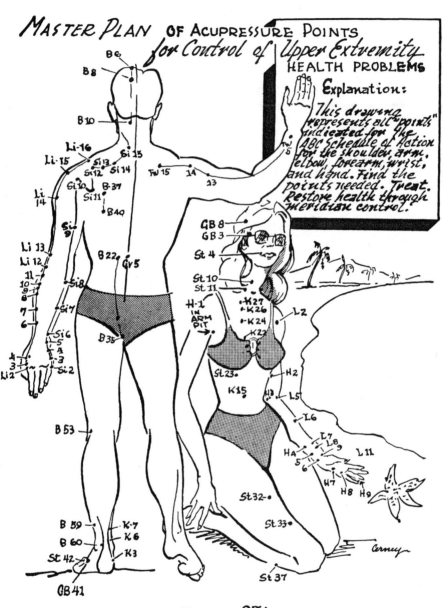

FIGURE 97A

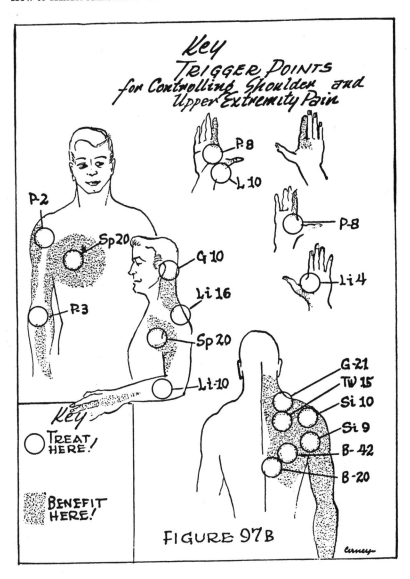

Key
TRIGGER POINTS
for Controlling Shoulder and
Upper Extremity Pain

P-8
L 10
P-8
Li 4
P-2
Sp 20
G 10
Li 16
P-3
Sp 20
Li-10

G-21
Tw 15
Si 10
Si 9
B-42
B-20

Key
○ TREAT HERE!

▓ BENEFIT HERE!

FIGURE 97B

Techniques for *The SHOULDER*

Procedure: Check your symptoms. Find the acupuncture points and acupress!

A B C SCHEDULE OF ACTION

SYMPTOMS	ACUPUNCTURE POINTS TO USE				
	A	B	C	D	E
Armpit swollen and painful	B-53	P-1	P-5	P-6	L-9
Arthritis	Si-3, 10 12	B-60	GB-3, 8, 41	St-4 42	Tw-5
Brachiitis (neuralgia)	K-27	L-2	Li-3, 4, 11, 14, 16	Si-2 13	B-10, 35, 40, 60
Bursitis	Li-10, 16	Gv-5.5	L-5	H-3	
Can't raise arm	L-2	Li-10, 12, 14, 16	H-1	Si-2, 9, 10	K-22
Capsulitis (frozen shoulder)	Tw-13	T-15	Si-11	Si-15	Li-16
Coldness	Si-14				
Hotness	Si-13				
Numbness	H-8	Si-40	Si-13		
Pain	L-6	Li-2	Li-12	Si-10	Si-14
Pain in "shoulder point" and arm	Li-15	B-6	B-37		
Rheumatism	B-8				
Spasm (muscle)	H-3	H-8	Si-7	Si-14, 16	B-35

Stiffness	T-14	B-22	
Swelling	Si-10		
Tension (muscles)	Si-10	Si-11	
Weakness	Si-10		

Techniques for *The UPPER ARM*

Procedure: Check your symptoms. Find the acupuncture points . . . acupress! (See Figure 97a.)

A B C SCHEDULE OF ACTION

SYMPTOMS	ACUPUNCTURE POINTS TO USE				
	A	B	C	D	E
Can't move arm backwardly	Tw-13	Li-16			
Can't raise arm	L-2	Li-10, 12, 14, 16	H-1	Si-2, 9, 10	K-22
Coldness	Si-14				
Coldness with spasms (muscles)	L-2,5	(Also see Figure 40)			
Hotness	L-2				
Loss of sensation	H-4	(Also see Figure 40)			
Neuralgia	Li-6	Li-7	H-5	Si-9	K-3
Numbness	Li-12				
Pain inside arm	P-2				
Paralyzed	Li-13	B-30	P-1		
Poor circulation	Li-10	(Also see Figure 40)			

Shaking (trembling)	L-9	(Also see Figure 40)		
Spasms (cramps)	L-10	H-5	Si-3, 7	P-7	Li-15
Swelling	K-7				

Techniques for *The ELBOW*

Procedure: Check your symptoms. Find the acupuncture points . . . acupress! (See Figure 97a.)

A B C SCHEDULE OF ACTION

SYMPTOMS	ACUPUNCTURE POINTS TO USE				
	A	B	C	D	E
Arthritis	H-4	Si-4			
Can't bend elbow	Si-7	H-6			
Pain with stiffness, muscle inaction, limited lifting of arm	Tw-13 15	Si-11	Si-15	Li-4	Li-16
Numbness	Li-12				
Spasm (muscles that control the elbow joint)	H-3		Tw-15	Si-11 15	Li-16

Techniques for *The FOREARM*

Procedure: Check your symptoms. Find the acupuncture points . . . acupress! (See Figure 97a.)

A B C SCHEDULE OF ACTION

SYMPTOMS	ACUPUNCTURE POINTS TO USE				
	A	B	C	D	E
Atrophy (shrinking of muscles)	St-32				
Can't raise arm	St-37	H-2, 3	Si-5	Si-6	B-59
Coldness	St-23	H-1			
Numbness	L-11	St-33	H-8	H-9	Li-9
Pain (neuralgia)	H-1, 2	H-4, 8	Si-5, 6, 11	K-3, 24	P-4
Paralysis of arm	H-1	Si-6	P-1		
Spasm (muscles)	H-2	Si-3	Si-4	Si-7	
Swelling	K-7				
Trembling	P-3 .				

Techniques for *The WRIST*

Procedure: Check your symptoms. Find the acupuncture points . . . acupress! (See Figure 97a.)

A B C SCHEDULE OF ACTION

SYMPTOMS	ACUPUNCTURE POINTS TO USE				
	A	B	C	D	E
Pain (neuralgia) wrist and fingers	Si-10	Si-11			

Stiffness	Si-10	Si-11, 15	Li-16	T-15	

Techniques for *The HAND*

Procedure: Check your symptoms. Find the acupuncture point ... acupress! (See Figure 97a.)

A B C SCHEDULE OF ACTION

SYMPTOMS	ACUPUNCTURE POINTS TO USE				
	A	B	C	D	E
Arthritis	H-4	Si-4			
Can't bend fingers	Si-4				
Can't hold anything	Si-7				
Coldness in hand	L-7	H-3	H-7	K-26	
Dulled sense of touch	Si-4				
Contractions (clawing)	H-8	P-8			
Frozen fingers	K-6				
Numbness	L-11	H-9			
Palms hot and painful	L-7	L-8	H-8		
Pain, with swelling	K-15				
Pain (neuralgia) in fingers	H-9	K-3	P-4	St-10	St-11
Spasm (muscles)	Li-15				

Stiffness	Pressure 1" and 4" lateral to thoracics 1 through 8			
Swelling (no pain)	K-7			
Trembling	Li-7	St-33	H-3	Si-8
Ulcer	Li-7			
Writer's cramp	P-8	B-10		

HOW TO HANDLE PAINS
OF THE BACK AND SPINE

7

$\mathbf{A}$ll back pains start with an initial irritant. The irritant may be anything. It may be as innocuous as a sneeze or as dramatic as diving off the cliffs into the water at Acapulco. These irritants affect the sensory nerves of the back and complications begin. These same nerves may be affected by bacteria, direct or indirect trauma, changes in temperature, chemistry foreign to the body, and even disease. Pain may be referred. There may be inborn malformations. Even more than this, there may be no existing physical problem yet the mind can play a disastrous role in pains of the back.

When you have a physical problem with your back, there are certain tangible signs and symptoms evident. Look for: bruises, discolorations, swellings, abnormal bony prominences, lumps or masses of foreign tissue, hips at different levels, foot problems and "broken arches," lesions in the spinal column, sacrum, and sacro-iliac joints, muscle tensions, and "knots" under the skin. All of them contribute to back pain.

NINE BASIC REASONS FOR
BACK MUSCLE PAIN

Pain in the back muscles may begin with: (1) *a direct blow and the reactive spasm*, (2) *indirect blows* (as in jumping from a height and landing on the heels), (3) *circulatory deficiency*, (4) *nutritional inadequacy*, (5) *abnormal tensions with emotional stress*, (6) *tensions from postural imbalance, congenital defects, and subluxated vertebrae causing nerve compression*, (7) *chilly drafts on sweaty back muscles* and weather change, (8) *twists and torsions* while in an awkward or unusual position, (9) *chest, abdominal, and pelvic organ disease* or impairment.

Each of these factors effectively influences the meridians and the acupuncture points that betray them. To give you a more precise understanding of the complexity of back problems, a number of illustrations follow. (See Figures 98, 99, and 100.) The brain and spinal cord are illustrated because the nervous system is so vital in acupuncture care. Note the direct connection between the spine and

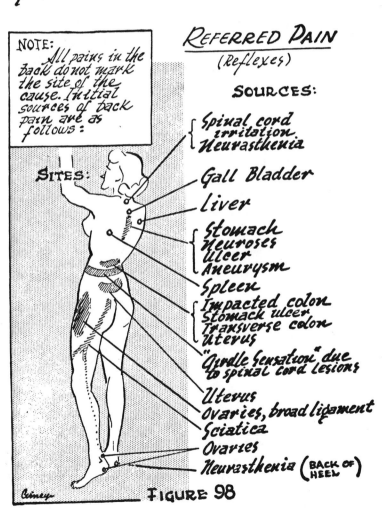

The BACK .... CATCH-ALL ..... for

NOTE:
All pains in the back do not mark the site of the cause. Initial sources of back pain are as follows :

REFERRED PAIN
(Reflexes)

SOURCES:

SITES:

{ Spinal cord irritation.
Neurasthenia

Gall Bladder

Liver

Stomach
Neuroses
Ulcer
Aneurysm

Spleen

Impacted colon
Stomach ulcer
Transverse colon
Uterus

"Girdle Sensation" due to spinal cord lesions

Uterus
Ovaries, broad ligament
Sciatica

Ovaries

Neurasthenia (BACK OF HEEL)

FIGURE 98

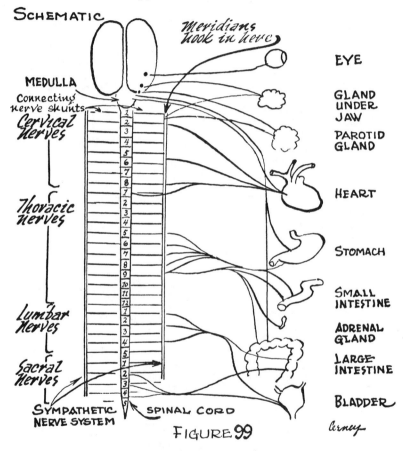

The SPINAL CORD - BRAIN- and SYMPATHETIC NERVOUS SYSTEM with which the Chinese meridians are intimately associated

SCHEMATIC

Meridians hook in here

EYE

MEDULLA

Connecting nerve shunts

Cervical nerves

GLAND UNDER JAW

PAROTID GLAND

HEART

Thoracic nerves

STOMACH

SMALL INTESTINE

Lumbar nerves

ADRENAL GLAND

LARGE INTESTINE

Sacral nerves

BLADDER

SYMPATHETIC NERVE SYSTEM   SPINAL CORD

FIGURE 99

Arney

the organs and parts involved. Note also how the sympathetic nervous system runs parallel to the spinal cord, and remember how the autonomic nervous system controls it all and how acupuncture points are the key to readjusting, rehabilitating, and renewing health in the tissues involved. Every Chinese meridian plays a role in this influence. Some of these meridians interlock, and what influences one influences them all. Like the lady with aching extremities said, "When your feet hurt, you hurt all over." And you do!

Note in Figure 98 that the causes of pain in the back have their origin removed from the point of where it seems to be occurring. Note too that when a spinal nerve is "cut off," damage to the part it feeds begins. These parts cry out through acupuncture points. They provide you with the key to your own therapy. They are Nature's way of saying, "X marks the spot!"

LUMBAGO

Lumbago is a dull, aching pain across the low back. From time immemorial, low back pain has plagued the human race, and only in the Orient did they have a way to cope with it successfully. From the Orient comes our Americanized *Acupressure, U.S.A.*, and how effective it is was noted in the case of teenager John Ray R., who was plagued with low back pain until acupressure was put to use.

Johnny injured his back seriously playing football. He couldn't raise himself up or turn over. He couldn't straighten. He couldn't even raise his leg without eliciting pain and anguish. He was given opiates and salicylates internally. He wore a plaster cast on his back and then a metal brace, and the agony went on until acupuncture and acupressure were used. But let's look at two other people with this same low back pain.

How the Agony of a Department Store Seamstress Was Relieved

In Janet R.'s case, her lumbago pain was of another origin. Janet's story was like so many heard before: doctors, drugs, multiple surgeries on her back and pelvis, and still the pain continued on. Her ovaries were gone. So were her uterus and appendix. Day after day, she went through the embarrassment and frustration of a colostomy bag for something the laboratory reported negative for cancer cells. She'd had x-rays and radium therapy and 18 sessions with a psychiatrist after she accused her physician of not knowing what he was doing. He exploded angrily and called her a goldbrick—and convinced that she *was* a goldbrick, she went to a head-shrinker just as she had been convinced by the surgeons that she needed surgery.

With Johnny, the high school football player, it had been a direct blow to his back that gave him pain. In Janet R.'s case, her lumbago-like pain turned out to be a kidney problem. She'd been treated for everything but the cause. *Symptoms and not the cause had been treated.* Nobody had stopped to check the acupuncture points that would have revealed her problem years earlier.

The Spinal Column ..... The Body Parts

..... when there is interference

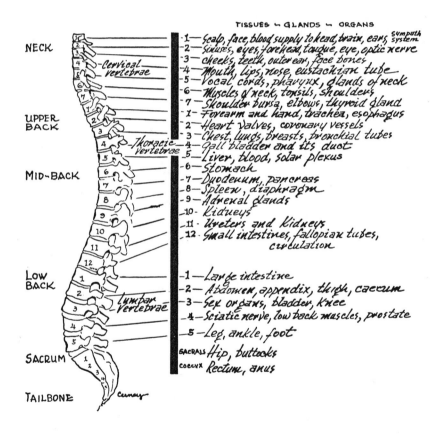

TISSUES – GLANDS – ORGANS

NECK

Cervical vertebrae

1 — Scalp, face, blood supply to head, brain, ears, Sympath system
2 — Sinuses, eyes, forehead, tongue, eye, optic nerve
3 — Cheeks, teeth, outer ear, face bones
4 — Mouth, lips, nose, eustachian tube
5 — Vocal cords, pharynx, glands of neck
6 — Muscles of neck, tonsils, shoulders
7 — Shoulder bursa, elbows, thyroid gland

UPPER BACK

Thoracic vertebrae

1 — Forearm and hand, trachea, esophagus
2 — Heart valves, coronary vessels
3 — Chest, lungs, breasts, bronchial tubes
4 — Gall bladder and its duct
5 — Liver, blood, solar plexus
6 — Stomach

MID-BACK

7 — Duodenum, pancreas
8 — Spleen, diaphragm
9 — Adrenal glands
10 — Kidneys
11 — Ureters and kidneys
12 — Small intestines, fallopian tubes, circulation

LOW BACK

Lumbar vertebrae

1 — Large intestine
2 — Abdomen, appendix, thigh, caecum
3 — Sex organs, bladder, knee
4 — Sciatic nerve, low back muscles, prostate
5 — Leg, ankle, foot

SACRUM

SACRALS Hip, buttocks
COCCYX Rectum, anus

TAILBONE   coccyx

FIGURE 100

ENERGIZED..... AILMENTS THAT MAY OCCUR

with nerve supply or Meridians

AILMENTS

Headaches, nervousness, insomnia, high B.P.
Deafness, earache, blindness, sinus trouble
Acne, eczema, neuralgia, neuritis
Allergies (hay fever), adenoids, catarrh
Laryngitis, hoarseness, "sore throat"
Tonsilitis, croup, stiff neck, pain in arms
Colds, goiter, bursitis
Asthma, cough, pain in forearm & hands
Heart problems, chest pain
Pleurisy, pneumonia, bronchitis, influenza
Gall bladder problems, shingles, jaundice
Liver problems, low B.P. anemia, arthritis
Stomach problems, indigestion, dyspepsia
Ulcers, diabetes, gastritis
Hiccough, stomach problems
Allergies, (hives etc)
Hardening of arteries, kidney trouble, tiredness
Acne, boils, eczema, auto-intoxication
Rheumatism, gas in bowel, sterility

Colitis, constipation, diarrhea, herniation
Cramps, acidosis, appendicitis, varicose veins
Bladder problems, knee pain
Lumbago, sciatica, pain or frequent urination
  (swelling)
Sudden legs & feet, poor circulation, coldness

Spinal curvature, sacro-iliac problems
Hemorrhoids, itching, pain on sitting.

Her *Kidney meridian* was hot, and as traditional Chinese doctors said, the kidneys control the fire of the Gate of Life. Deficiency of kidney *yang* caused the spleen *yang* to be deficient. *Ch'i* departed from the heart and it started to palpitate. Weakness of lung *ch'i* produced difficulty in breathing, and because of *yang* emptiness she sweated spontaneously. The body tried to tell the doctors all this, but they did not listen. No one had stopped to use the Oriental wisdom of yesterday that points out how all such symptoms and signs exhibited by Janet were the result of kidney insufficiency.

A Little Old Man Is Cured of Lumbago

Willie had periodic low back pain. His lumbago was an acquired characteristic. When I arrived on the family scene the first time, Willie was piled high with hot water bottles and electric blankets . . . the worst thing in the world for a back problem of any kind . . . and there he lay in agony.

His family doctor had pronounced the problem "lumbago" two weeks previous and gave him a pain killer. After two weeks, the pain continued. No effort had been made to determine whether the problem was of bacterial or viral origin or even if it was truly lumbago. No effort was made to check Willie's history or his physical anatomy. No one paused to remember Willie's wartime injury or that his problem was postural due to a surgically shortened leg. With the pelvis tilted and the spine scoliotic, Willie's muscles were in a state of spasm. They remained that way until acupuncture and acupressure were used. I had them slide a piece of plywood under Willie's mattress to keep his back from sagging, and a pillow under his knees to relieve muscle tension, and then ran a differential diagnosis to determine if my diagnosis was right—and by the time the treatment was completed, Willie was asleep. The thigh injury he received going over-the-top of the trench in the Argonne Forest disaster of World War I gave him a permanent reminder of his problem.

Other Causes of Low Back Pain About Which You Must Be Cautioned

In dealing with low back problems, there are a number of

factors to remember: (1) any *infection or inflammation within the body* may manifest itself as back pain (for example, fever diseases); (2) *pain originating in the abdomen or pelvis may refer to the low back* (for example, colitis, a sagging large bowel, prostate and urethral diseases, ovary and uterus problems—all or any of them may trigger pain in the back. Backaches may begin with kidney stones and cystitis); (3) *postural problems*; (4) *direct and indirect injury* are other causes.

In Willie's case it wasn't even *lumbago*. It was his "short leg" kicking up the fuss in his low back. Part of the thigh bone had been shot away, and surgical help created a structural difference leading to twisting and torsion of the tissues above.

Then there was Jeff J. Jeff was a middle-aged man bowed down with family responsibilities. He was a cement finisher. He had a low back problem that every doctor in our town had treated at one time or another. Jeff went to the hospital obediently for surgery on his back for a "slipped disc." He took all the drugs prescribed and stuck to the rules, but the low back pain continued. When I first saw Jeff, he was in abject misery. Two sons carried him in. After complete x-ray studies and examination, the problem was obvious. It was a congenital malformation of the fifth lumbar vertebra. The ten-dollar word for it is *spondylolisthesis*, and acupressure and acupuncture admittedly were temporarily useless. Only manipulation of this forwardly subluxated bone would bring relief. This was done. Today Jeff walks in peace.

What I am saying is don't expect Acupressure, U.S.A. to be a panacea. There's nothing in the world that is. DO expect, however, little miracles of your own that you can create day after day, little miracles that get rid of low back pain in the following manner:

A B C SCHEDULE OF ACTION
for LUMBAGO

A	B	C	D	E	F	G
B-30	GB-4	Si-17	Sp-2 8 19	L-5	Li-4	See the "Z" zones of the foot (Fig. 23)

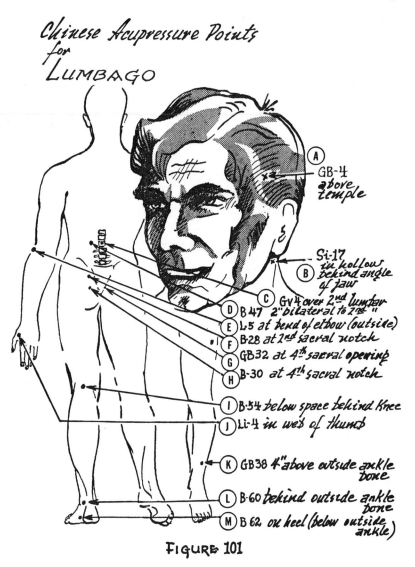

Chinese Acupressure Points
for
LUMBAGO

(A) GB-4 above temple

(B) Si-17 in hollow behind angle of jaw

(C) Gv4 over 2nd lumbar

(D) B47 2" bilateral to 2nd "

(E) L5 at bend of elbow (outside)

(F) B28 at 2nd sacral notch

(G) GB32 at 4th sacral opening

(H) B-30 at 4th sacral notch

(I) B-54 below space behind knee

(J) Li-4 in web of thumb

(K) GB38 4" above outside ankle bone

(L) B-60 behind outside ankle bone

(M) B 62 on heel (below outside ankle)

FIGURE 101

Supplementary
Procedures

1. *Physical therapy.*

(a) *Icepacks* on "trigger points" of pain. *No heat!* (Physiological fire is already raging in lumbago. Objective is to cool it and put it out.)

(b) *Massage* all muscles of the back and thighs gently but firmly.

(c) *Coldpacks* from mid-back down to base of spine.

    Procedure: (after second day)

        1. Coldpack for 15 minutes.

        2. Hotpack for 15 minutes.

        3. Coldpack for 30 minutes. Alternate or repeat three times. This will make you drowsy, so just go to sleep.

2. *Remove the cause!*

3. *Improve faulty posture.*

4. *Exercise* to strengthen the back muscles. (Use corrective procedures indicated in Figure 102.)

Low Back Corrective Exercises

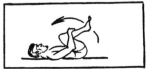

LYING ON ABDOMEN
Raise head, arms and legs high.

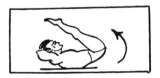

LYING ON ABDOMEN
Clasp hands behind back. With legs down raise head and torso.

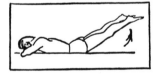

LYING ON ABDOMEN
Face down on folded arms. Raise legs high behind you.

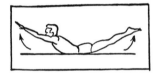

LYING ON BACK
Lock hands behind head. Bend at middle. Bring legs up.

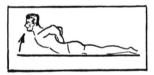

LYING ON BACK
Knees to chest. Hold. Return. Rest. Repeat.

Amey FIGURE 102.

LOW BACK CORRECTIVE EXERCISES (Figure 102)

NOTE: *Continue exercises in Figure 102 as long as necessary and remember that in lying on your back—and rocking back and forth—you are rendering Acupressure to the acupuncture points of your back.* These exercises may be used in all low back problems *after* the inflammatory and spasm stage has eased up.

SACRO-ILIAC PAIN

Sacro-iliac pain is that pain usually found on one side of the low back and extending down the sciatic nerve into the extremity.

In addition to direct injury to the above-named joints, there are a number of other causes for sacro-iliac pain. Broken arches may contribute to pelvic distortion. Pregnancy and too much lying in bed may be a causative factor. Subsequent attacks may follow such trivial matters as sneezing or the more gross effect of lifting and twisting. It may start with getting up out of bed or out of a soft easy chair. Faulty posture is a contributing agent. Pain, in this condition, is accentuated by lifting the leg on the affected side. Bending at the waist, or leaning sideways or forward, may aggravate it.

This is the way it was with Major Haley whose problem began just by turning at the waist while demonstrating a wall chart. Pain shot down his back and thigh. It was a disabling pain, and he came to the office in a wheel chair. In turning to his audience, he actually—and with no pre-meditated aforethought—pushed the upper portion of his sacrum forward, stretched the joint, the sacral nerves, and the lumbo-sacral cord. Treatment was rendered, and he took home a little chart showing the following Schedule of Action:

A B C SCHEDULE OF ACTION
for Sacro-Iliac Pain

A	B
B-28	GB-27
29	30
60	

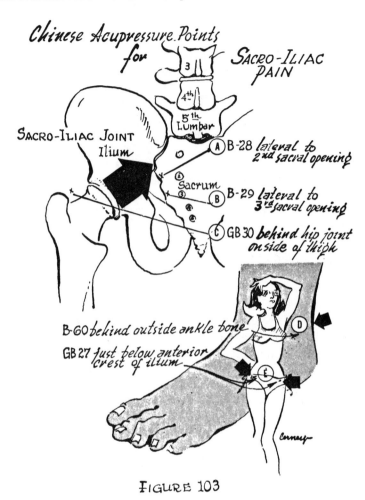

Figure 103

Supplementary
Procedures

1. *Physical therapy.*

(a) Sleep with pillow under knees and one under the low back.

(b) Massage muscles of the low back and thigh. *Do not* massage over the sore joint.

(c) Coldpacks over the sore joint for the first two days. Thereafter, use hotpacks if the pain persists.

(d) Supportive bracing is temporarily helpful.

SCIATICA

Sciatica is inflammation of the sciatic nerve trunk, with concurrent pain extending as far down as the foot as it becomes more chronic.

For example, when Kate L. had her first baby, she began losing the ability to use her left leg. X-rays of Kate's pelvis revealed the head of the fetus putting pressure on the sciatic nerve area. After delivery, the pain went promptly away. Old John R.'s leg "went dead" when his prostate enlarged. Bookkeeper Layne S. got it from being cocked on the edge of his chair all day. Race driver Danny L. got "automobile sciatica" every time he made a speed-run over 100 miles long. The point is that *pressure triggers the problem.*

In the joint-disease form of sciatica, any involvement of adjacent bones may trigger it off. In sciatic neuritis, the pain is usually on one side only. It may burn, stab, or feel like it's being ripped. Pain more often is in the back of the thigh. Sometimes it is confined to the outside of the leg, the area behind the knee and the foot. *Anyone who has the problem can put his finger right on it, and each one of these trigger zones of pain is an acupuncture point!*

Hypersensitive areas may be located in the middle of the thigh (B-51), in the sciatic notch of the pelvic bones (B-48), at the fifth lumbar vertebra (Gv-2.3), the crest of the ilium in back (B-47), at the outside ankle bones (B-60), and in the popliteal space (B-54) behind the knee. The accent on sciatica is pain relief, and this is accomplished in the ABC Schedule of Action that follows. The second move is "Find the Cause!"—because no matter what treatment you render, if the original irritant remains, you will get a re-occurrence of the problem over and over.

A B C SCHEDULE OF ACTION
FOR SCIATICA

A	B
B-47	Gv-2
48	3
51	
54	
60	

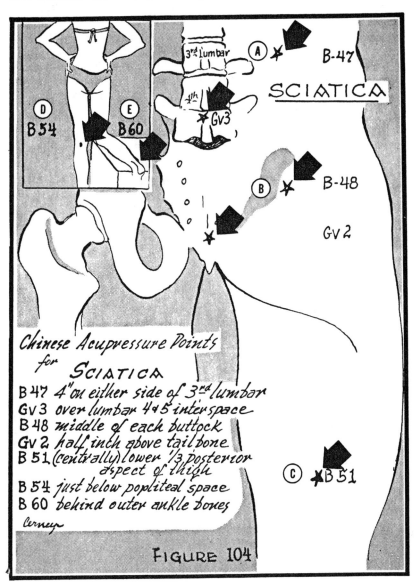

Chinese Acupressure Points
for SCIATICA

B 47 4" on either side of 3rd lumbar
Gv 3 over lumbar 4 & 5 interspace
B 48 middle of each buttock
Gv 2 half inch above tailbone
B 51 (centrally) lower 1/3 posterior
          aspect of thigh
B 54 just below popliteal space
B 60 behind outer ankle bones

Cerney

FIGURE 104

**Supplementary
Procedures**

NOTE: Treatment varies with whether the sciatic problem is acute (having it for the first time) or whether it has happened before (chronic). All supplementary procedures are based on these stages:

Acute Stage:
  1. *Physical therapy.*
      (a) *Coldpacks* along the course of the affected nerve, even while maintaining general body warmth with blankets.
      (b) *Immobilize the limb* with pillows, with one pillow under the knee.
      (c) *Use your fist as a fulcrum*, to be placed under your low back—knuckles up—at the originating point of pain. Lie on this wedge for five minutes.
  2. *Dietary controls.*
      (a) Rich foods, unless rheumatism or gout preclude this type of diet.
  3. *Bowels.*
      (a) Keep bowels purged daily if inactive.

Chronic Stage:

  1. *Physical therapy.*
      (a) *HOT applications* followed by cold to stimulate circulatory reaction. Keep leg active while submerged in tub.
      (b) *Mild massage*—but *not* over the sciatic nerve or other painful areas. Begin active nerve stretching by gently extending the leg. REMEMBER: Chronic or acute—*find the cause!* Prevent it from happening again!

BONUS THERAPIES

NOTE: A full page illustration follows on Acupuncture pressure points to use in *treating back pain.*

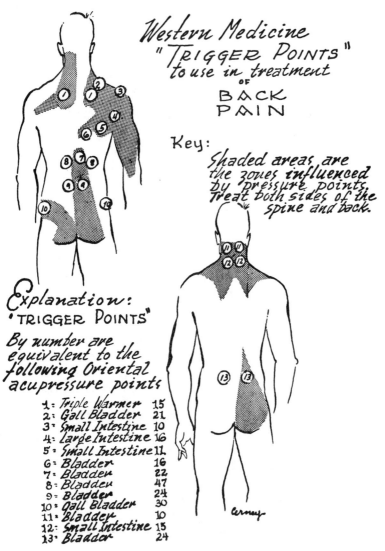

Western Medicine
" TRIGGER POINTS "
to use in treatment
OF
BACK
PAIN

Key:

Shaded areas are
the zones influenced
by pressure points.
Treat both sides of the
spine and back.

Explanation:
'TRIGGER POINTS"

By number are
equivalent to the
following Oriental
acupressure points

1= Triple Warmer   15
2= Gall Bladder   21
3= Small Intestine 10
4= Large Intestine 16
5= Small Intestine 11
6= Bladder   16
7= Bladder   22
8= Bladder   47
9= Bladder   24
10= Gall Bladder   30
11= Bladder   10
12= Small Intestine 15
13= Bladder   24

FIGURE 105

THE CARE OF SEX ORGANS
FOR A MORE DYNAMIC SEX LIFE

8

ACUPRESSURE "BOOSTER SHOTS"
FOR MORE DYNAMIC MALE SEX LIFE

Acupressure, U.S.A. has proven of infinite value to those men complaining of impotence, lack of virility, and "loss of manhood." Some men account for their problem as being due to some childhood infection such as mumps. Some indicate a blow to the crotch. Others honestly admit that it's a state of mind.

John G., an architect with a flair for the dramatic, complained of lost potency, that he couldn't copulate, that he was sterile, barren, and that it was making serious inroads into his career as well as his life. He asked woefully what was left in life once a good, clean sex life was gone.

I told him the best answer to his problem was *Acupressure, U.S.A.* I explained how autonomic controls of the nervous system could help him build a more dynamic sex life, that after the initial office treatment, he could follow an ABC Schedule of Action by himself at home. In using these amazing Oriental secret procedures, "the old order would changeth and youth would spring up once more." By pressing the right acupuncture buttons, sexual pleasure and marriage relationship would be enhanced and made to come alive once more!

If you would improve *your* sexual performance, as did John G., in just a few weeks, use the following acupressure "booster shots" that will change the course of your life.

How to Improve Your Sex
Life via Acupressure, U.S.A.

1. *Testicular Compression.* Grasp the scrotum and its contents

202

gently in one hand. Apply firm on-off pressure 25 times daily.

2. *Perineal Pressure Points.*

(a) This "hot spot" is located between the scrotum and the anus. It is at this point that the "Conception Vessel," as named by the Orientals, begins. Acupuncture point *Cv-1 is a stimulation center.* It's indeed a "hot spot" on yourself and on the female.

(b) Now make pressure around the rim of the anus.

(c) Locate Gv-1. This is the key sex-stimulating center found equidistant between the anus and the tip of the coccyx (tail bone). Press. repeat five times. Release. All gently.

3. *Symphysis Pubes Contact.* Just below the hair line, where the right and left pubic bones meet, is a key area of stimulation. To the left and right of the symphysis pubes are additional zones. In using acupressure on these zones, you are stimulating the *Spleen, Stomach, Kidney,* and *Conception Vessel meridians* on a horizontal plane. Apply rotary pressure on separate points that are on inch intervals out from the central midline (Sp-12, St-29, K-12, and Cv-3).

4. *Abdominal Organ Stimulation.* Ailing internal organs inhibit sex life. They destroy libido when you're sick and worn out. Because of this, it is vital that you . . .

(a) *Relieve constipation.* Use fingertip pressure on the navel.

(b) *Stimulate the liver.* Cup the fingertips of both hands up under the edge of the right rib cage. Press. Relax. Breathe deeply and repeat (five repetitions).

(c) *Solar plexus pressure.* Press the fingertips of both hands into the area below the tip of the sternum (breastbone). Hold. Relax. Breathe deeply and repeat again (five repetitions).

5. *Lower Lumbar Pressure Technique.* With hands on hips and thumbs projecting backwardly, insert the thumbs into the hollow on each side of the spinal column. Press deeply. Release. Repeat on the lower three lumbar vertebrae (five repetitions).

6. *Medulla Oblongata Technique.* Here's the grand finale to each day's treatment. The medulla oblongata is the master tuner-upper. It is the dynamo for vitality, the sex-stimulator, and all you have to do is insert the third finger of each hand into that magic hollow at the base of the skull. Press. Release. Relax. Repeat five times.

Use this procedure daily for best results. The few moments you spend with this sex secret from the Orient will restore your sex vitality.

PROSTATE PROBLEMS

The *prostate* gland in the male is a part-glandular, part-muscular body surrounding the proximal end of the urethra and the neck of the bladder. It is about the size of a horse chestnut and frequently enlarges in the middle years to close off urination.

About 40 per cent of the males over 60 have an enlarged prostate. Half of these men experience no problems. In some individuals, the enlargement may be due to tumors. But no matter what the initial cause, when enlargement takes place, it contributes to bladder infection, dilatation of the bladder, retained urine, formation of intestinal infection, and bladder stones. It may even contribute to high blood pressure and septic poisoning by interfering with the urination of watery waste. There may often be an urgency to urinate, and yet the urine won't come. Sometimes this feeling is just a false alarm. Sometimes when the stream is voided, the urine burns. The stream may get feeble so that the bladder is never emptied at any one time and this very fullness is a source of irritation.

A Prostate Patient's Case

I remember a gentleman we'll call "Old Joe." Old Joe walked the quarter mile from the nursing home down to my office. His blood pressure was up and he was mentally confused. Uremia was poisoning him. His heart was compensating. He said he couldn't get any sleep because he spent the night running to the toilet. Prostatic obstruction wasn't as yet complete, but urine was already backing up through the cesspool system.

Trigger points at the ankle were given treatment. So were others that you will note in the ABC Schedule of Action. (See also Figure 106.) He was given a copy of these instructions and told to administer his own therapy. He did. Old Joe dialed the phone himself. He was very pleased. He was no longer walking around disorientated. Apparently, the uremia and self-poisoning were gone. The night-time urination had stopped. Urgency, frequency, and smarting were no more.

A B C SCHEDULE OF ACTION
FOR PROSTATE PROBLEMS

A	B	C	D	E	F	G
Sp-6 15	Cv-1 4 6 7	K-5 7 27	Liv-9	Gv-1	B-31 32 65	Prostate "Z" zone on foot

IMPOTENCE

Impotence is the inability of the male to achieve erection to participate in sexual intercourse. By any name, impotence is a mind-rattling problem with a lot of men, and the inability to have an erection marks a mental disaster area that may shape the course of their lives. Orientals, dealing in this area with acupuncture, have found that when the truly impotent male has this problem, his anxiety subsequently affects his heart and his spleen. When a male has a healthy desire for intercourse, but has to suppress it, this constant repression finally affects his liver. Of the 145 impotent Chinese men treated by one researcher, 137 were restored to their former manliness.

A Truck Driver's Cure

Mental hang-ups are, in most part, responsible for the majority of male impotency cases. With this in mind, it is still necessary for the doctor to make a thorough examination of glands, checking for previous infections or illnesses and diseases of the genitalia. Of the many causes contributing to impotency, there was the case of Pete W. Pete was a taxi driver. Prior to that, he drove a truck. Taxi and truck drivers are subject—because of their long sitting—to *traumatic prostatitis*. In Pete's case this was the problem. In that male gland was the key to his impotency. To conquer it, the following acupuncture points were used via *Acupressure, U.S.A.*, and today Pete's mighty proud of himself. He's had three children by his third wife! (See also Figure 107.)

Chinese Acupressure Points
for

PROSTATE
PROBLEMS

Sp 6 *On angle of jaw*

K·27 *below head of*
clavicle

Sp 15 *abdomen - on level*
with umbilicus
Cv 7 *one inch below "*
Cv 6 *two inches " "*
Cv 4 *three " " "*
Cv 1 *symphysis pubes*
B 31 *over 1st sacral opening*
B 32 *over 2nd " "*
Gv 1 *tip of tailbone*
Liv-9
NOTE: *Also see "Z" zones*
in foot for "Sex Glands"

K·7 *above inside ankle*

K-5 *behind inside ankle*
bone
B-65 *lateral side of foot*

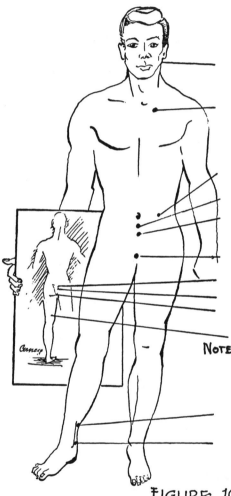

FIGURE 106

A B C SCHEDULE OF ACTION
FOR IMPOTENCE

A	B	C	D	E	F	G
K-2 10 12	B-15 31 32 35 38 47 49	Sp-6	Cv-2 6	L-7	St-30	H-8

(See Figure 107)

SPERMATORRHEA

Spermatorrhea—traditionally called "wet dreams"—is a nocturnal emission of sperm with or without dreams.

In watching one Oriental physician's approach to five different men with the problem, I saw—as he asked questions and used the meridians and tender acupuncture points for guides—that the problem with these men was more of a physical nature rather than emotional.

In one case, the patient's face was pale, emaciated, his pulse weak. Another patient showed heart palpitations, complained of insomnia, weakness, and no appetite. His face also was haggard. The third couldn't get his thinking coordinated. His pulse was empty. The fourth and fifth men were fat and they too had no appetite. Their pulses were deep. Although each was different from the other, the same acupuncture and acupressure procedure was successfully used. Here are the pressure points you can use in your own home. See Figure 108.

A B C SCHEDULE OF ACTION
FOR SPERMATORRHEA

A	B	C	D	E
Sp-2 6 8 9	Cv-3 4	St-36	B-12, 15 21, 23 31, 38 47, 50 67	K-12

(See Figure 108)

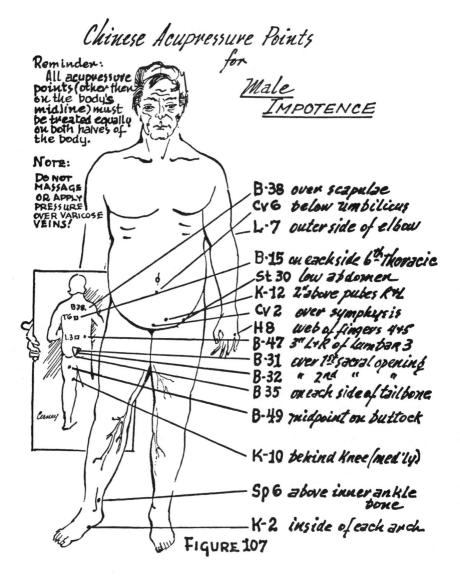

Chinese Acupressure Points for

Male IMPOTENCE

Reminder:
All acupressure points (other than on the body's midline) must be treated equally on both halves of the body.

NOTE:
DO NOT MASSAGE OR APPLY PRESSURE OVER VARICOSE VEINS!

B-38 *over scapulae*
Cv6 *below umbilicus*
L-7 *outer side of elbow*

B-15 *on each side 6th Thoracic*
St 30 *low abdomen*
K-12 *2" above pubes R+L*
Cv 2 *over symphysis*
H8 *web of fingers 4+5*
B-47 *3rd L+R of lumbar 3*
B-31 *over 1st sacral opening*
B-32 *" 2nd " "*
B 35 *on each side of tailbone*

B-49 *midpoint on buttock*

K-10 *behind knee (med'ly)*

Sp 6 *above inner ankle bone*

K-2 *inside of each arch*

FIGURE 107

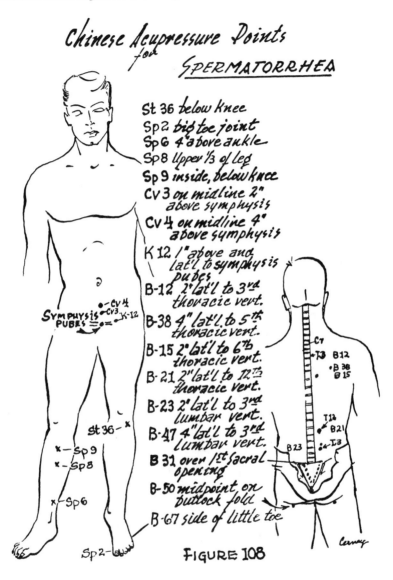

Chinese Acupressure Points for SPERMATORRHEA

St 36 *below knee*
Sp 2 *big toe joint*
Sp 6 *4" above ankle*
Sp 8 *Upper 1/3 of leg*
Sp 9 *inside, below knee*
Cv 3 *on midline 2" above symphysis*
Cv 4 *on midline 4" above symphysis*
K 12 *1" above and lat'l to symphysis pubes*
B-12 *2" lat'l to 3rd thoracic vert.*
B-38 *4" lat'l to 5th thoracic vert.*
B-15 *2" lat'l to 6th thoracic vert.*
B-21 *2" lat'l to 12th thoracic vert.*
B-23 *2" lat'l to 3rd lumbar vert.*
B-47 *4" lat'l to 3rd lumbar vert.*
B-31 *over 1st sacral opening*
B-50 *midpoint on buttock fold*
B-67 *side of little toe*

Symphysis Pubes

FIGURE 108

BONUS THERAPIES (Figures 109-113)

	A	B	C	D
Frigidity	K-7	St-29	Sp-16	Cv-4

	A	B	C	D
Lack of Desire	Liv-8	Si-5	Tw-4	Gv-1, 2

	A	B	C	D
Male Sterility	Sp-5	B-32 33	K-5	Tw-10

	A	B	C	D
Pain in Penis	L-7	St-29 30	Sp-6	B-47 50

	A	B	C	D
Premature Ejaculation	B-23	Li-4	Tw-10	K-5

ACUPRESSURE "BOOSTER SHOTS"
FOR WOMEN ONLY!

Sexual response and more glorious living through "feeling like a woman again," is possible through secrets long hidden in the Orient and now made available to you through *Acupressure, U.S.A.* You *can* stay younger and live longer! You *can* have those added years of sex life that mean so much to a woman when she feels she's "going downhill." To help you in this matter, I brought back from the Orient eight techniques—"booster shots"—that could very possibly change the course of your life!

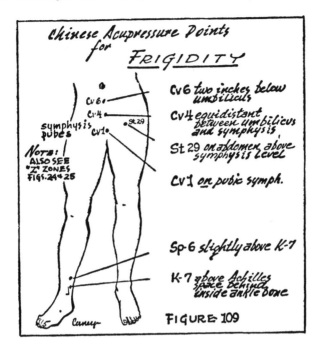

Chinese Acupressure Points for FRIGIDITY

Cv6 *two inches below umbilicus*

Cv4 *equidistant between umbilicus and symphysis*

St 29 *on abdomen, above symphysis level*

Cv1 *on pubic symph.*

Sp-6 *slightly above K-7*

K-7 *above Achilles space behind inside ankle bone*

symphysis pubes

Note: Also see "Z" Zones Figs. 24 & 25

FIGURE 109

Acupressure, U.S.A. . . . the
Key to Sexual Awakening

Here's how to do it:

1. *Teach the male.* Let him know where your most erogenous sexual zones are! Oriental women, schooled to please, utilize this method frankly and with intent.

2. *Thumb pressure on lower lumbars.* With arms akimbo and hands planted on hips, insert your thumbs into the hollows at either side of the lumbar vertebrae. If you have a fat pad at this point and you are not getting through, either lie on your fist or a golf ball at these key points. Repeat on the sacrum.

3. *Solar plexus pressure.* Take advantage of an important plexus of nerves at this point by applying the fingertips of both hands. Press just below the tip of the sternum (breastbone). Release. Press deeply. Hold. Relax. Breathe deeply and repeat (five repetitions).

4. *Titillation of the nipples.* The tips of the breasts mark a highly sensitive acupuncture point. This is St-17 of the *Stomach meridian*, and you can use it to your advantage day after day. Not

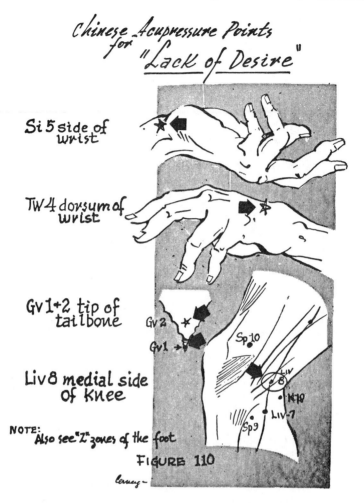

Chinese Acupressure Points for "Lack of Desire"

Si 5 side of wrist

TW 4 dorsum of wrist

Gv 1+2 tip of tailbone

Gv 2

Gv 1

Sp 10

Liv 8 medial side of knee

LIV 8

K 10

LIV 7

Sp 9

NOTE: Also see "Z" zones of the foot

FIGURE 110

Carney-

just to stimulate sexual desire but to build your breasts and bring them erect. Stimulate by rubbing or other procedure.

5. *Thyroid stimulation.* Pressure on acupuncture points on the neck are very important as a "booster shot" for sex stimulation. The most important is S-10. This important point not only steps up sex reaction but capability as well.

6. *Inguinal area sensitivity.* Place the hands, palms down, at the point where the thighs meet the body. Press. Repeat five to ten times.

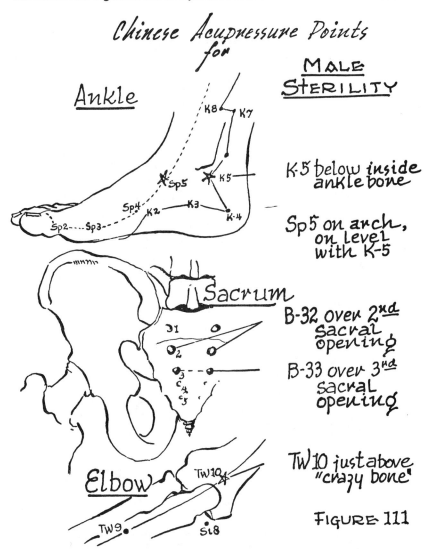

Chinese Acupressure Points for

MALE STERILITY

Ankle

K-5 below inside ankle bone

Sp 5 on arch, on level with K-5

Sacrum

B-32 over 2nd sacral opening

B-33 over 3rd sacral opening

Elbow

TW 10 just above "crazy bone"

FIGURE 111

7. *Medulla oblongata pressure.* Third finger of each hand into the hollow at the midline base of the skull. Rotate fingertips until tenderness is gone.

8. *Massage the breasts.* Palms down, make massagic motions, circling from the inside, down, around, with the breasts cupped in the hand, and pulling up gently. Repeat ten times.

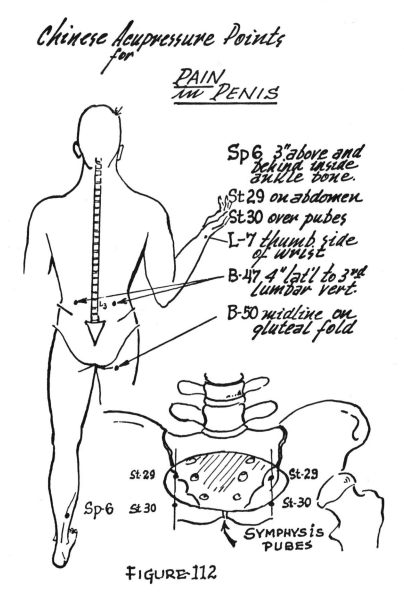

Chinese Acupressure Points
for

PAIN
in PENIS

Sp 6 3" above and behind inside ankle bone.

St 29 on abdomen

St 30 over pubes

L-7 thumb side of wrist

B-47 4" lat'l to 3rd lumbar vert.

B-50 midline on gluteal fold

St-29   St-29
Sp-6   St-30   St-30

SYMPHYSIS PUBES

FIGURE 112

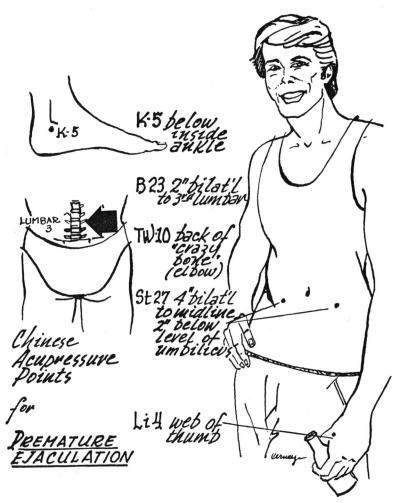

K-5 below inside ankle

B 23 2" bilat'l to 3rd lumbar

TW 10 back of "crazy bone" (elbow)

St 27 4" bilat'l to midline, 2" below level of umbilicus

Li 4 web of thumb

Chinese Acupressure Points for PREMATURE EJACULATION

FIGURE 113

NOTE: *The following six feminine problems are very personal problems that play a delicate and sometimes indelicate role in the lives of women. The Oriental approach to gynecology is different from ours in Western-style medicine. Yet, I've watched it succeed when Western-style medicine failed or rendered only partial relief. Acupuncture, and Acupressure, U.S.A., may very possibly be YOUR answer to a feminine matter that has long been a problem to you!*

MENOPAUSE

Menopause, as the Oriental defines it in calling it *Yin Lian*, is that moment in her life when a woman ceases to be able to bear children.

In a day of dramatically harsh drug-interference with the capability for conception—and the trail of disaster that it is leaving in its wake—the birth control "pill" has changed this definition in the 20th Century, and the role that it will play in the future has the aura of a vast question mark around it.

Although menopause is said to be a normal consequence of the passage of years, it doesn't fit that pattern for all women. Some women never even know they have passed into the stage of infertility . . . it goes by so gently. Others live through a unique kind of feminine hell that causes problems for everyone around them, and, in most part, the problem is self-imposed! Then, there are those who go on into the older years still active sexually, still bearing children, and everyone marvels.

Under normal circumstances, somewhere between the ages of 45 and 50, the ovaries decline in their function of releasing fertilizable ova (eggs). The menstrual period ceases, gets scant, or goes like crazy in what the girls call "flooding." It's a period of problems of one kind or another, and they are all due to endocrine imbalance caused by some instability in the autonomic nervous system . . . that system so beautifully controlled by acupuncture and *Acupressure, U.S.A.*

If ovarian regression is slow, a woman may experience none of the "change of life" symptoms. But where ovarian function stops abruptly, the symptoms of the climacteric are strong and shattering, with flushes, chills, excitability, and anger coming out of nowhere, crying spells, depression, forgetfulness, tiredness, dizziness, headaches, tingling, joint pain, backache, itching, sweating, heart palpitations, urinary inadequacies, abdominal difficulties—a host of problems besetting her all because her ductless glands (thyroid, adrenals, pituitary, ovaries) are functioning inadequately.

Because Acupressure, U.S.A. deals in the autonomic nervous system which influences these key ductless glands, it is the procedure of choice in coping with this feminine problem that causes so many women so many ungracious moments in their lives.

If *you* are having such a problem, use *Acupressure, U.S.A.*! Use it to advantage. Use the God-given controls that Nature has already given you. Use those acupuncture points that contain the very secret of Oriental wisdom. Use them to help smooth out that period of "change of life"—which comes to men as well as women—with the passage of the years.

A Maiden Lady Solves the
Rigors of "Change of Life"

Laura J. was a sweet little woman. She was just four-foot-eleven, had never married, supported her mother and invalid sister, and had dedicated her life to them.

Off and on again, she had the works—delinquent menstrual periods and sometimes "flooding," flushes and chills, depression, backaches, crying spells, headaches, dizziness, tingling, heart palpitations, and frequent desire to urinate. It was all there—a train of problems on the annoying track of growing older, signs and symptoms a doctor must analyze because too often the same problems may result from organic as well as psycho-genic causes.

After complete examination I told her I wasn't certain what the results would be, but since she had already run the gamut of "estrogenic shots," and all the rest from her M.D., with only temporary relief, then acupressure was worth the gamble.

Laura made the gamble. We used *Acupressure, U.S.A.* and also worked the reflex areas of her feet. A week later, she returned to the office. I was astonished. The bent-over little old lady I'd seen the week previous had been transformed! She was standing erect! Her shoulders were back, breasts held high in health and pride, and her face was glowing. I couldn't believe my eyes, but there she was reporting that she was sleeping every night—which she hadn't done in months—that there had been no recurrence of hot flashes or chills. She said, "I feel like living again!" Apparently *Acupressure, U.S.A.* changed the course of her life, because the following month she was married!

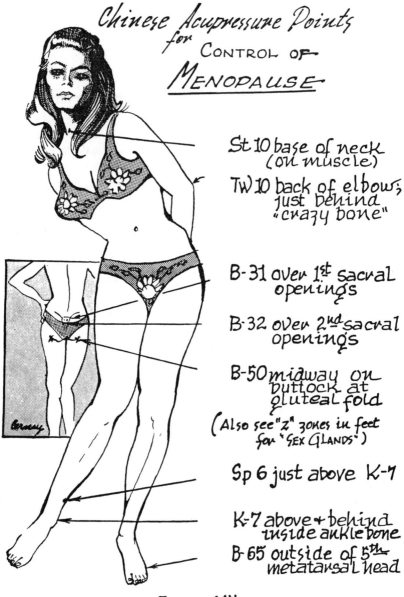

Chinese Acupressure Points for CONTROL OF *MENOPAUSE*

St 10 base of neck (on muscle)

Tw 10 back of elbow; just behind "crazy bone"

B-31 over 1st sacral openings

B-32 over 2nd sacral openings

B-50 midway on buttock at gluteal fold

(Also see "z" zones in feet for "SEX GLANDS")

Sp 6 just above K-7

K-7 above + behind inside ankle bone

B-65 outside of 5th metatarsal head

FIGURE 114

A B C SCHEDULE OF ACTION
FOR MENOPAUSE

A	B	C	D	E	F
Sp-6	B-31 32 50 65	St-10	K-7	Tw-10	"Z" zones (for ovary, pituitary, thyroid) in the foot (See Fig. 23)

IRREGULAR MENSTRUATION

That which the Chinese called *"Yue Fing By Tiao"* (irregular menses) has long been a problem with women who are otherwise healthy and yet worry immeasurably when their "period" is not on time. A very nice lady with this problem was Janet D. She was married, 28, and didn't want any more children than the three she already had. When her menstrual irregularity began, she naturally thought she was pregnant again, and this started a war at home.

She took her problem to her neighborhood physician, who said it was glandular, that what she needed was thyroid control even though her basal metabolism test was normal. Then he tried her on cyclic courses of male hormones when the thyroid tablets didn't work. Following that came estrogen (female hormone) "shots." Following that came combinations of estrogen-progesterones, and her problem persisted.

Because it had become a family problem, Janet asked me one day about the matter. We discussed her obviously clean bill of health as being quite different from those women who had irregular menstrual periods as the result of hidden infections, glandular or organic disorders, etc. She wanted a course of corrective action. The following schedule was suggested, and within three months her periods were on a 28-day cycle once more. See Figure 115.

A B C SCHEDULE OF ACTION
FOR IRREGULAR MENSES

A	B	C	D
Sp-4	Cv-3	St-25	B-23
6	4	33	32
8	6		
10			

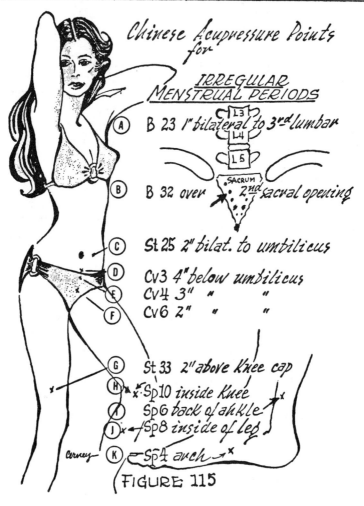

Chinese Acupressure Points for

IRREGULAR MENSTRUAL PERIODS

(A) B 23 1" bilateral to 3rd lumbar

(B) B 32 over 2nd sacral opening

(C) St 25 2" bilat. to umbilicus

(D) Cv3 4" below umbilicus
Cv4 3" " "
Cv6 2" " "

(G) St 33 2" above knee cap
(H) x Sp10 inside knee
(I) Sp6 back of ankle
(J) Sp8 inside of leg
(K) Sp4 arch

FIGURE 115

PRURITIS VULVAE

Pruritis vulvae is that irritating local itch of the vulva (the external part of the female's genital organs). This embarrassing problem was given the name of *"Yin Yang"* by the Chinese. Its source and its treatment is often difficult to single out. Melanie M. had this persistent itch for months, and it got so bad that she was ready to explode emotionally. When she phoned my office for an appointment, she was crying. She said the itching was so bad that she couldn't even control her urine and had to change her underthings a half-dozen times a day. After trying all the doctors in town, she landed in my office. My suggestion, "Well, you've tried everything else, let's give *Acupressure, U.S.A.* a whirl." She did. It worked! Here's the procedure we used. See Figure 116.

A B C SCHEDULE OF ACTION
FOR PRURITIS VULVAE

A	B	C	D	E	F	G
Sp-6 10	Liv-2 11	B-54 60	Cv-1 3	St-30	Gv-1	H-8

(See Figure 116)

Supplemental Procedures

1. *Physical therapy.*
   a. *Icepack* one hour per day over sacral area.
   b. *Massage* and loosen all muscles of the low back (three times per week).
2. Maintain hygienic cleanliness.

LEUKORRHEA

Leukorrhea is often called "the whites" and is a non-bloody discharge from the vagina that is aggravating and annoying to the female.

Usually it is an infection in the vagina or cervix that causes "the whites," which the Chinese call *"Dai Xai."* Many factors lower the resistance of this organ so that fungus, bacteria, or protozoa make their invasion of this private track. A patient of mine we'll call Mabel

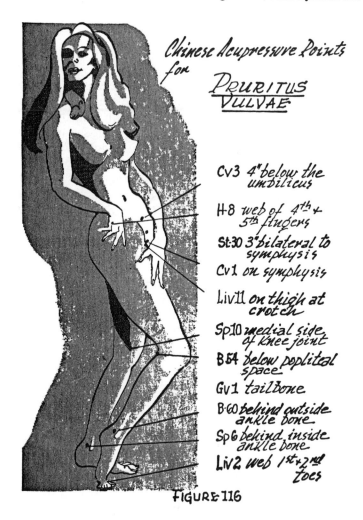

Chinese Acupressure Points for

PRURITUS VULVAE

Cv3 *4" below the umbilicus*

H-8 *web of 4th + 5th fingers*

St-30 *3" bilateral to symphysis*

Cv1 *on symphysis*

Liv11 *on thigh at crotch*

Sp10 *medial side of knee joint*

B54 *below popliteal space*

Gv1 *tailbone*

B-60 *behind outside ankle bone*

Sp6 *behind inside ankle bone*

Liv2 *web 1st + 2nd toes*

FIGURE 116

M. said she had had her "whites" since childhood, that her undergarments had been soiled as far back as she could remember, that her vulva was red, swollen, and slick. At puberty she still had it, and the annoyance carried through into adulthood. That's when she got married and her husband picked up the same thing. It was this explosive moment that sent her in to see me. After ruling out all possibilities via laboratory and examination, Chinese therapy was begun. Here are the acupuncture points that "cleared up" the whole problem.

A B C SCHEDULE OF ACTION
FOR LEUKORRHEA

A	B	C	D	E	F	G
B-31 32 33 44	GB-26	St-25	Cv-3	Sp-6 8 9	H-6 9	All "Z" zones in the foot (Fig. 23)

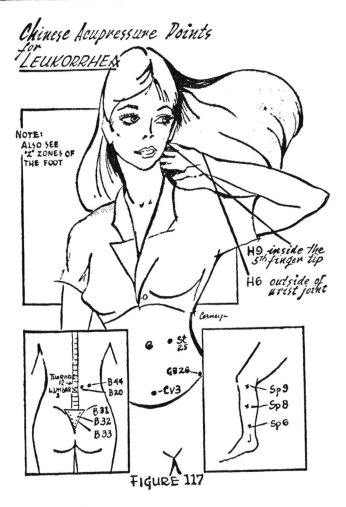

Chinese Acupressure Points for LEUKORRHEA

NOTE:
ALSO SEE
"Z" ZONES OF
THE FOOT

H9 inside the 5th finger tip

H6 outside of wrist joint

Cerney—

St 25

GB 26

Cv3

Thoracic 12 →
LUMBAR 1

B 44
B 20

B 31
B 32
B 33

Sp 9
Sp 8
Sp 6

FIGURE 117

Supplementary
Procedures

  1. *Physical therapy.*
      a. *Coldpacks* from midback to end of spine, 30 minutes daily.
      b. *Massage* to loosen up all back muscles.
      c. *Stay off feet.* Rest.
      d. Use douches only as a cleansing agent.
  2. *Contraindications.*
      a. Don't exert yourself.
      b. Stop worrying about everything!

AMENORRHEA

Amenorrhea is the total absence of the menstrual period from any cause. In most part, it is the *Bladder meridian* that is offended. In Western-style medicine pre-mature menopause is blamed on the lack of proper hormones. Undeveloped uterus, ovarian failure, and lack of thyroid are said to be causative factors. The pituitary and adrenals may play an intimate role. Stress is also laid on malnutrition, systemic disease, obesity, and diabetes. Western medicine utilizes a "shotgun" approach with hormones and hopes that one of them gets through to do the trick. The Oriental acupuncturist points out a more specific route.

A B C SCHEDULE OF ACTION
FOR AMENORRHEA

A	B	C
B-20	Cv-3	St-29
21, 23	4	30
37, 38		36

Supplementary
Procedures

  1. *Physical therapy.*
      a. *Massage* to loosen all muscles of the low back. Get them totally relaxed. This will also affect all the Chinese meridians that control the pelvic area.

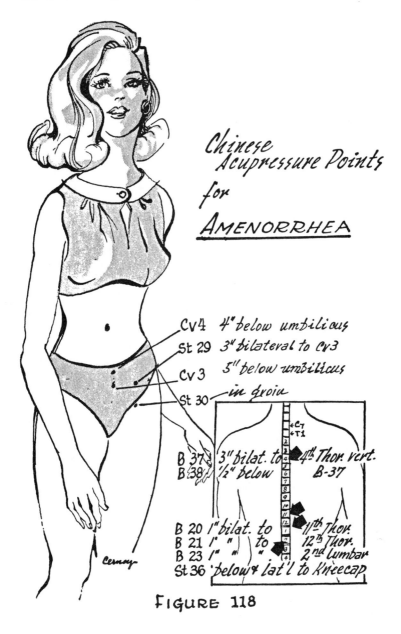

Chinese
Acupressure Points
for
AMENORRHEA

Cv4   4" below umbilicus
St 29   3" bilateral to Cv3
Cv 3   5" below umbilicus
St 30   in groin

←C7
←T1

B 37   3" bilat. to   4th Thor. vert.
B 38   ½" below   B-37

B 20   1" bilat. to   11th Thor.
B 21   1"   "   to   12th Thor.
B 23   1"   "   "   2nd Lumbar
St 36 below & lat'l to Kneecap

Cerney

FIGURE 118

  b. *Heat applications* daily over lower dorsal, lumbar, and
sacral regions.
  c. *Warm vaginal irrigations.* Temperature 90°F. Five-
minute treatment.
2. *Contraindications.*
  a. Avoid too much study, overwork.
  b. Don't get cold and damp.
  c. Don't permit poor health to get you down. Eat right.
Sleep enough. Get outside for exercise.

DYSMENORRHEA

Dysmenorrhea is painful menstruation for which there may or
may not be any apparent cause. Teenager Marjory H.'s pain started
with cramps in her lower abdomen. Pain extended up into her back
and down her thighs just before her period. She'd had it ever since
her periods began at age 14. Her folks gave permission for a physical
and pelvic examination, and outside the fact that she wasn't a virgin
any longer, there was no evidence of any underlying pelvic or
systemic condition. I told her parents privately that usually after
young ladies were married, and had their first child, the problem
disappeared. In the meantime, suggestions were made for current
comfort for this painful menstrual problem the Chinese call *"Tong
Fing."* After treatment there was no return of pain.

A B C SCHEDULE OF ACTION
FOR DYSMENORRHEA

A	B	C	D	E	F	G	H
H-5	St-24	Liv-13	Cv-4	B-23	Sp-9	K-2	Gv-12
	25	14	6	31	10	3	
				17		6	
				62		13	

Supplemental
Procedures

  1. *Physical therapy.*
    a. *Massage* all muscles of the low back.
    b. *Icepack* over the lumbar and sacral region. Place hot
water bottle on lower abdomen.

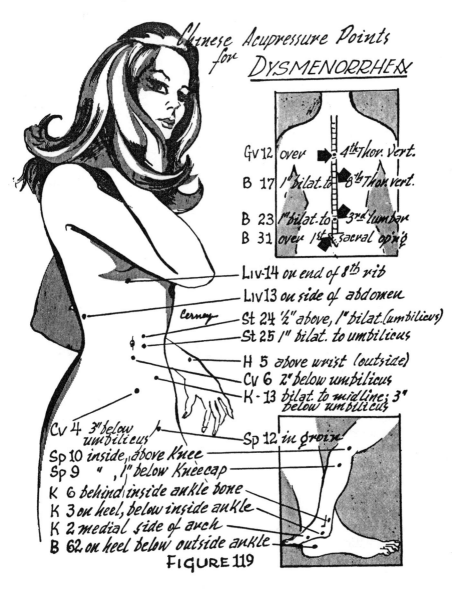

Chinese Acupressure Points
for DYSMENORRHEA

Gv 12 over → 4th Thor. Vert.
B 17 1" bilat. to 8th Thor. vert.
B 23 1" bilat. to 3rd lumbar
B 31 over 1st sacral op'n'g

Liv-14 on end of 8th rib
Liv 13 on side of abdomen
St 24 ½" above, 1" bilat.(umbilicus)
St 25 1" bilat. to umbilicus
H 5 above wrist (outside)
Cv 6 2" below umbilicus
K-13 bilat. to midline; 3" below umbilicus

Cv 4 3" below umbilicus
Sp 12 in groin
Sp 10 inside, above knee
Sp 9 " , 1" below kneecap
K 6 behind inside ankle bone
K 3 on heel, below inside ankle
K 2 medial side of arch
B 62 on heel below outside ankle

FIGURE 119

    c. *Hot water footbath.*
2. *Food control.*
    a. *Wholesome diet* with Vitamin E supplement.
3. *Exercise.*
    a. Daily walks between periods.
    b. Rest in bed during the "period."

4. *What to avoid.*
   a. Getting chilled. (Keep feet and legs warm.)
   b. Sexual excesses.
   c. Tight bands around the waist.
   d. Fatigue and nervous tension.
5. *Important point to remember.*
   a. When *Acupressure, U.S.A.* brings no relief, you are on the wrong acupuncture points, or,
      (1) If pain begins *before* the flow, there is an ovarian involvement.
      (2) If pain begins *with* the flow, it indicates some involvement of the uterus.

THE GENITO-URINARY SYSTEM

Cystitis (Bladder, Inflammation of)

Cystitis is an inflammation of the urinary bladder caused by bacteria, or their toxins (poisons), to medication, food, or direct injury.

Cystitis may be acute or chronic. In the acute form, urination may be painful and interrupted. There may be dribbling day or night. In the chronic form, there may be pain during urination. There may be pus in the urine. A policewoman with this problem came to see me about it. She was a strong-minded woman who asked questions but didn't listen to answers. I explained to her how infections may ascend up into the bladder by way of the urethra, and how they may descend into the bladder by way of the ureters and kidneys or from other organs nearby, that there are many pre-disposing causes, and none of them are simple, that with cystitis, pain may precede, accompany, or follow urination. Policewoman Johannsen indicated that her urination terminated with a succession of painful spasms, that sometimes there was constant pain deep in the pelvis, with some of it radiating upward into the abdomen and some of it radiating down the thigh. In addition to pus, I found blood in her urine. She said that the bleeding occurred at the end of the urination. Examination and further tests revealed nothing. When asked about activities, Miss Johannsen admitted studying karate. She remembered taking a kick "down low in the breadbasket!" Here's the acupressure program I laid out for her.

A B C SCHEDULE OF ACTION
FOR CYSTITIS

A	B	C	D	E
Cv-2 3	B-32 54 65	Gv-1	K-8	St-30

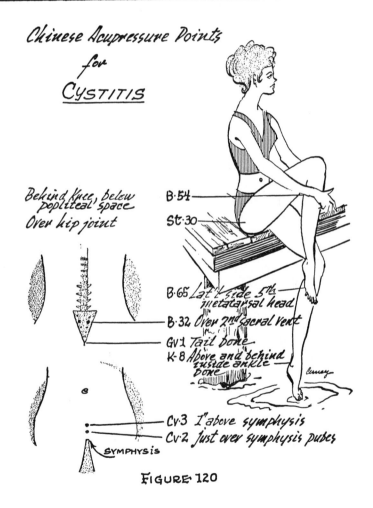

Chinese Acupressure Points
for
CYSTITIS

Behind Knee, below
poplicteal space
Over hip joint

B·54

St·30

B·65 Lat'l side 5th
metatarsal head

B·32 Over 2nd sacral vent

Gv1 Tail bone

K-8 Above and behind
inside ankle
bone

Cv·3 1" above symphysis

Cv·2 Just over symphysis pubes

SYMPHYSIS

FIGURE 120

**Supplementary
Procedures**

1. *Physical therapy.*
   a. *Rest in bed.* Elevate hips.
   b. *Coldpacks* over lumbar and sacral areas (low back). Where this does not bring relief with acupressure procedures, follow with an ice water enema and then hotpacks over the bladder.
   c. *Massage* the abdomen deeply but gently.
2. *Dietary supplements.*
   a. *Light diet* only (soups).
   b. *Drink a lot of water.* Peppermint tea is excellent.
   c. *Keep the bowels open* by refraining from starches and protein solids.

Enuresis
(Bed Wetting)

In the adult, urinary enuresis should not be confused with *incontinence* (an explanation of which follows later). An individual may be born with a weak "sphincter." He may develop or acquire the problem. Usually the condition starts around age five or six. Bed wettings have many causes. They may range from improper training to hypo-thyroidism, from mental defects to internal problems. Local irritation that brings on the desire to urinate may stem from such problems as fissures, polyps in the rectum, vulvo-vaginitis in the female, too acid or too concentrated urine, or too great an ingestion of liquids. Pinworms may be a contributing problem. It may occur in children as the result of malnutrition, anemia, tuberculosis of the bladder, inherited tendencies, or even from insecurity. In all cases training is necessary, and acupressure treatment has to be designed to eliminate the cause and diminish the irritability that triggers it.

ABC SCHEDULE OF ACTION
FOR BED WETTING

A	B	C	D	E	F
Cv-1	Liv-4	K-5 10	G-33	B-34 51 65	Si-8

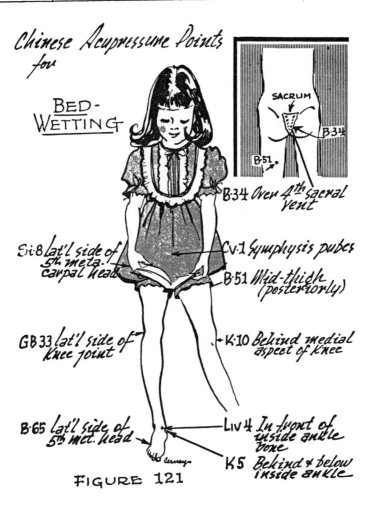

Chinese Acupressure Points for

BED-
WETTING

SACRUM

B-34

B-51

B-34 Over 4th sacral vent

Si-8 lat'l side of 5th meta-carpal head

Cv-1 Symphysis pubes

B-51 Mid-thigh (posteriorly)

GB 33 lat'l side of knee joint

K-10 Behind medial aspect of knee

B-65 lat'l side of 5th met. head

Liv 4 In front of inside ankle bone

K-5 Behind & below inside ankle

FIGURE 121

Supplementary
Procedures

    1. *Physical therapy.*
        a. *Cold applications* to be applied on the lower thoracic area and lumbar vertebrae for 30 minutes before bedtime. Twice weekly.
        b. *Elevate the foot of the bed.*
        c. *Cold footbath* before retiring. Follow with brisk towel rub.
    2. *Dietary control.*
        a. Eat largest meal at noontime. Light dinner. Avoid all salts and sweets after 4 PM.

I found the following additional acupressure point procedure of value to an electric power lineman who developed bed wetting after receiving a large jolt of electricity on the job. These are the instructions he followed.

Technique:

    (a) *Thumb pressure in the lumbar area.* With the thumbs, compress the areas on either side of the lumbar vertebrae.
    (b) *Compress pressure points over the sacrum.*
    (c) *Probe the reflex areas of the foot* as indicated in the attached diagram.
    (d) *Abdominal pressure.* Apply abdominal pressure with the palms while in a lying down position. Then apply the same pressure centrally over the bladder.
    (e) *Solar plexus pressure.* Place all fingertips in the area and press. Hold for a three count and relax. Repeat five times.
    (f) *Medulla oblongata pressure.* Place the third finger of each hand in the hollow at the base of the skull. Use rotary pressure until all tenderness is gone. Finish with . . .
    (g) *Coldpack on the belly.* And go to sleep!
    (h) *The Award System.* When used on children, should take the place of threats, spankings, or other reprimands. With "nervous" children don't permit them to get fatigued before retiring. Teach them to evacuate before bedtime. Reward them for their good results. At no time chastise them!

Urinary Incontinence

Incontinence is the uncontrolled loss of urine—"stress leakage"—that has nothing to do with sleep. It is a common gynecological complaint. Ranging from "dripping" to uncontrolled "free flow," it has its beginnings somewhere in the bladder or urethra. Childbearing, sex relations, injury such as from horse or bicycle riding, over long periods of time, may contribute to the problem.

Mrs. Rena J., housewife and mother of five children, developed urinary incontinence when she least wanted it. One daughter was getting married, one graduating from high school, the other was at the hospital having a baby, and Mrs. J. ran the entire route and dripped all the way. Her complaint was that it began after re-arranging the living room furniture. From that time on, it occurred when she carried heavier packages, picked up the grand-children, walked up or down steps, or even when she got excited about something. Her clothing was immediately stained.

What happened was that with the rise of emotions, anger, frustration, there was an instant increase in intra-abdominal pressure!

Intra-abdominal pressure places stress on the urinary bladder. Compressing it promotes leakage. Stress causes it to let loose, and Mrs. J.'s children were prompt to notice it. They complained of the odor that clung to her at all times, and it was embarrassing to everyone concerned. She stopped going shopping. She wouldn't attend her husband's office parties or go near people, and here she was involved now with all her daughters at very crucial moments in their lives when they needed their Mom.

Mrs. J. complained that along with the leakage, she also had a peculiar feeling of "something dragging" or "something loose" down there (lower vaginal area).

Examination revealed nothing complicated. The ABC Schedule was used. (See also Figure 122.) Since that time Mrs. J.'s family no longer teases her about carrying along her own emergency pot. Utilizing the Chinese pressure points, the dripping has stopped, and Mrs. J. has gone back to being with people once more.

A B C SCHEDULE OF ACTION
FOR URINARY INCONTINENCE

A	B	C	D	E	F	G
Sp-11	H-5 8	B-21 30	Cv-3 4	St-36	K-14	See "Z" zones in feet (Fig. 23)

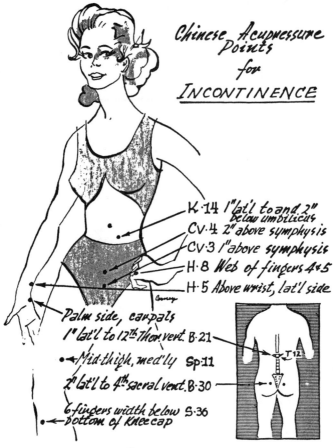

Chinese Acupressure Points for
INCONTINENCE

K·14 *1" lat'l to and 2" below umbilicus*
Cv·4 *2" above symphysis*
Cv·3 *1" above symphysis*
H·8 *Web of fingers 4 & 5*
H·5 *Above wrist, lat'l side*

Palm side, carpals
1" lat'l to 12th Thor. vert. B·21
Mid-thigh, med'ly Sp·11
2" lat'l to 4th sacral vert. B·30
6 fingers width below bottom of kneecap S·36

T·12

FIGURE 122

Nephritis

Nephritis is simply inflammation of the kidney due to bacteria, their toxins, or other poisonous waste.

Nephritis comes in two varities: *acute* and *chronic*. The acute form involves little filtration units in the kidneys called *glomeruli*, the tubules, and finally the entire organ. Various parts of the kidney may be involved simultaneously.

Toxic drugs such as alcohol, arsenic, mercury, etc. may cause the problem. Diphtheria, septicemia, scarlet fever, may trigger it. Exposure to cold and wet, and even malnutrition, may bring it on.

How Winnie W. Overcame Nephritis

Winnie W. came into my office complaining of headache, weakness, digestive disturbances, dry skin, and the fact that she was having trouble with her vision. She complained about her fingers getting white and tingly, and that she was dizzy, nauseated, and constantly tired. Sometimes she was even stuporous, and the problem got so bad she had to quit her job. Everything was happening to this poor woman.

Mrs. W.'s blood pressure was way up. She cried about how she urinated constantly. Her urine sample was low in specific gravity when tested. It also showed albumin and cysts. Blood samples revealed urea, uric acid, and creatinine. The dear lady was markedly anemic, pale, and insecure. Her eyelids were nearly swollen shut. With her morale at its deepest low, we went to work. Hygienic and dietetic procedures were laid out for her. With the ABC Schedule that follows, she recovered within weeks, and the last time I saw her on the street she reported, "Everything's OK." See Figure 123.

A B C SCHEDULE OF ACTION
FOR NEPHRITIS

A	B	C	D	E
G-25	B-22 25, 54 62	St-18 36	Sp-13	K-1 5 7 10

(See Figure 123)

Supplementary
Procedures

1. *Physical therapy.*

a. *Hotpacks* on lower thoracic vertebrae and upper lumbars. Half hour twice daily. After improvement starts, use hotpacks three times weekly, but increase treatment time to one hour per session.

b. *Hot baths* twice weekly. Remain in hot tub *only* until such time as the sweat breaks out on your forehead.

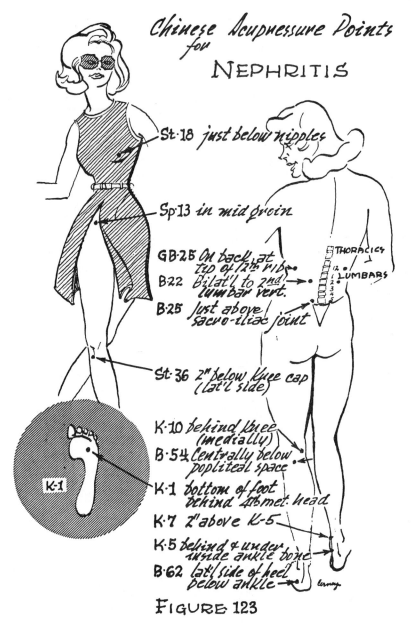

Chinese Acupressure Points for NEPHRITIS

St·18 *just below nipples*

Sp·13 *in mid groin*

GB·25 *On back, at tip of 12th rib*

B·22 *Bilat'l to 2nd lumbar vert.*

B·25 *Just above sacro-iliac joint*

THORACICS
LUMBARS

St·36 *2" below knee cap (lat'l side)*

K·10 *behind knee (medially)*

B·54 *Centrally below popliteal space*

K·1 *bottom of foot behind 1st met. head*

K·7 *2" above K-5*

K·5 *behind & under inside ankle bone*

B·62 *lat'l side of heel below ankle*

K-1

FIGURE 123

c. *Massage* all back muscles and down over the sacrum. Massage the adbomen deeply but gently.

2. *Regular outdoor exercise.*
3. *A dry, warm climate is best.*
4. *Wear enough clothing to maintain body warmth.*
5. *Dietary controls.*
    a. *Light diet* (soup) with a lot of other liquids. *No meat!* To this diet, add stewed prunes, baked apples, orange juice, rice pudding. Drink plenty of milk if you can tolerate it.

    AVOID: all seasoned foods, pastries, alcohol, tea, coffee, spices, drugs.

    DO USE: corn bread, tapioca, rice, macaroni, fresh vegetables, butter, bacon, potatoes, olive oil, white meat of chicken, fresh fish, clams, fresh beef, young mutton, buttermilk, ginger ale, lemonade, oranges, apples.

NOTE: When the kidneys are functioning inadequately, there is a lessened desire for sex life. The person with nephritis gets tired and timid. His neck gets tense. He has trouble with his vision. He has earaches. Most of all he has no push—and K-10, with the other acupuncture points, will help you conquer all this. K-1, 5, and 7 will give you more drive and ability "to go."

Urine Retention

Urine retention is the failure or inability to expel urine from the bladder, and thus contributes to problems that afflict the genito-urinary system.

Mrs. Preston wasn't young. She wasn't old either. But one thing that complicated her life was the fact that she couldn't urinate. properly. Her bladder had simply lost tone because she was anemic, and according to her story there were a number of other problems that aggravated the situation. One was the fact that if anyone was in the same bathroom with her, she simply couldn't expel. When she was nervous about something, it got worse. Exposure to cold weather multiplied the problem, and very apparent was the fact that the nerve endings in the bladder simply weren't responding. The condition began as a post-operative complication. Mrs. Preston catheterized regularly after her operation for a retroverted uterus, and the bladder wall simply became inactive. It looked like another trip to surgery until her relatives suggested acupuncture and *Acupressure, U.S.A.* . . acupuncture without needles that was not only simple to apply but relieved her problem. Here are the control buttons she pressed. See Figure 124.

A B C SCHEDULE OF ACTION
FOR URINE RETENTION

A	B	C
Sp-9, 10, 11 12	B-48, 54, 65	Cv-2, 9

Chinese Acupressure Points for The RETENTION OF URINE

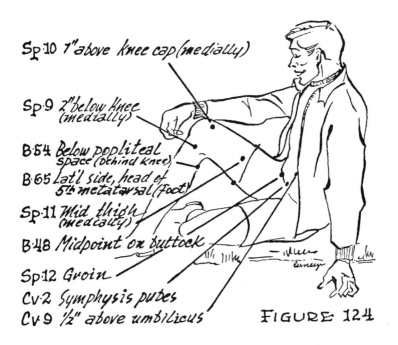

Sp-10 *1" above knee cap (medially)*

Sp-9 *2" below knee (medially)*

B-54 *Below popliteal space (behind knee)*

B-65 *Lat'l side, head of 5th metatarsal (foot)*

Sp-11 *Mid thigh (medially)*

B-48 *Midpoint on buttock*

Sp-12 *Groin*

Cv-2 *Symphysis pubes*

Cv-9 *½" above umbilicus*

FIGURE 124

HOW TO HANDLE
GASTRO-INTESTINAL AND
ABDOMINAL PROBLEMS

9

Abdominal Pains
(What They May Be Telling You)

When pains occur in the abdomen, they are too often complex and deceitful, and a little time must be spent here to give you an awareness of why drugs and surgery are often no answer to the problem.

Pain in the abdomen may be the result of local malfunction or disease. It may be visceral and diffuse itself in all directions. It may come from some somatic (muscle or bone) source, and as such be confined in one area. However, here's the number one point that even doctors sometimes forget: *That abdominal pain may be stemming from another body part!* Figure 125 gives you the rundown on this connection.

WITH PAIN FROM ANY CAUSE,
HERE'S THE AMAZING PHENOMENON
ABOUT ACUPRESSURE CARE

It is true that intra-abdominal pain may come from gastro-intestinal problems such as appendicitis, hernia, peptic ulcer, or even diverticulitis. It may stem from hunger, overeating, or a dozen other local problems. It may come from some problem in the genito-urinary system, from the pancreas, liver, or gall bladder. It may come from the peritoneum. But even more then this, it may have its inception in another body part; example—the heart.

239

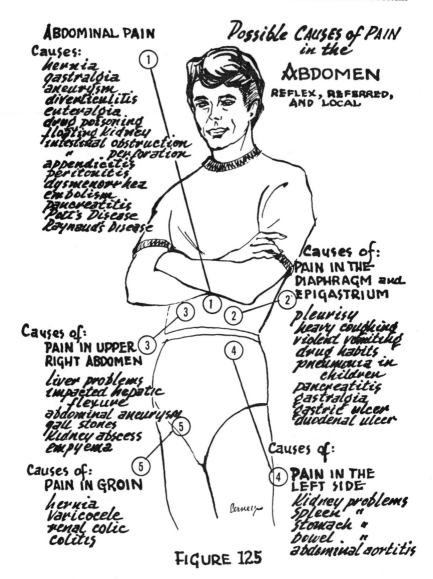

ABDOMINAL PAIN

Causes:
hernia
gastralgia
aneurysm
diverticulitis
enteralgia
drug poisoning
floating kidney
intestinal obstruction
"   perforation
appendicitis
peritonitis
dysmenorrhea
embolism
pancreatitis
Pott's Disease
Raynaud's Disease

Possible Causes of PAIN in the **ABDOMEN**

REFLEX, REFERRED, AND LOCAL

Causes of:
PAIN IN THE DIAPHRAGM and EPIGASTRIUM

pleurisy
heavy coughing
violent vomiting
drug habits
pneumonia in children
pancreatitis
gastralgia
gastric ulcer
duodenal ulcer

Causes of:
PAIN IN UPPER RIGHT ABDOMEN

liver problems
impacted hepatic flexure
abdominal aneurysm
gall stones
kidney abscess
empyema

Causes of:
PAIN IN GROIN

hernia
varicocele
renal colic
colitis

Causes of:
PAIN IN THE LEFT SIDE

kidney problems
spleen   "
stomach   "
bowel   "
abdominal aortitis

FIGURE 125

The heart, like other extra-abdominal organs, may refer its hurt into the abdomen, and even for a doctor this often leads to confusion and demands tests and examinations to determine cause. Knowing and treating the cause is vital to self-preservation, but *one of the amazing factors about acupuncture and Acupressure, U.S.A. is that it doesn't always matter what the cause is!* If you have located and relieved the right acupuncture point, the organ or part with which it is associated rights itself, and the pain disappears automatically!

Pain may be referred *in* the abdomen from the spinal nerves, the lungs, the spinal bones, sickle cell anemia, syphilis, and even from drug withdrawal, and have nothing to do with the gastro-intestinal organs themselves! By treating the right meridians, therefore, Nature does the job. By autonomic nerve stimulation, or even sedation, these organs, or parts, are alleviated of their distress.

**You Don't Have to Be
a Doctor to Conquer
Self-Help Problems**

APPENDICITIS

A B C SCHEDULE OF ACTION

(Mild Appendix Problems Only)

NOTE: Don't gamble with appendicitis symptoms. Life is too important. It's even more important than your convictions, so put the problem in your doctor's hands. He's better prepared to handle the matter than you are.

A	B	C	D	E	F
St-21 36	Si-8	B-22 63 Right foot side of spine only	K-3 11	XL-3	The "Z" zones of the foot (Fig. 23)

(See Figure 126)

**Supplementary
Procedures**

1. *Physical therapy.*

a. *Coldpacks* over lumbar area when there is pain. Also cover lower thoracic vertebrae. When pain subsides, use heat on

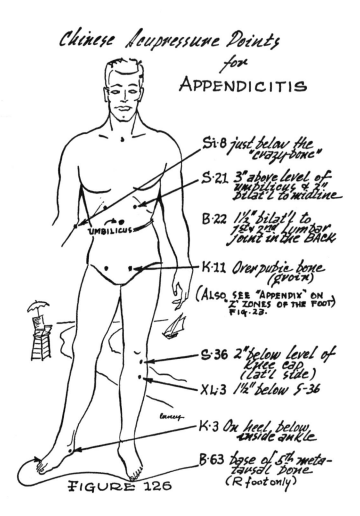

Chinese Acupressure Points for
APPENDICITIS

Si·8 *just below the "crazy-bone"*

S·21 *3" above level of umbilicus & 2" bilat'l to midline*

B·22 *1½" bilat'l to 1st & 2nd lumbar joint in the BACK*

UMBILICUS

K·11 *Over pubic bone (groin)*

(ALSO SEE "APPENDIX" ON Z' ZONES OF THE FOOT) FIG·23.

S·36 *2" below level of knee cap (lat'l side)*

XLi·3 *1½" below S-36*

K·3 *On heel below, inside ankle*

B·63 *base of 5th metatarsal bone* (R foot only)

FIGURE 126

abdomen (solar plexus area as well as over appendix area). Utilize hotpacks. Repeat daily till distress is gone.

    b. *Warm soapsuds enema* to relieve the lower bowel of foreign material. *Do not take a laxative!*

    c. *Massage* the muscles of the low back, upper back, and neck. *Do not massage over the abdomen!*

2. *When in doubt, see your doctor immediately!*

COLITIS

Colitis—also called "irritable colon"—is a functional disorder involving the intestines, with diarrhea alternating with constipation as a common complaint.

Although specific causes of colitis are unknown, it is deemed by Western medicine to be due to (a) *bacteria*, (b) *allergies*, and (c) *emotions*. Ulcerative colitis may occur at any age but usually hits in the second, third, and fourth decades of man's life. It may start slowly and leave no mark, or be acute and demonstrate itself with diarrhea or watery stool, lost appetite, slight temperature rise (usually at night), sometimes nausea and vomiting. There may be some abdominal tenderness, but it seldom leaves any external physical signs other than possibly hemorrhoids and external itching of the anus. Your ABC's to handle this matter are as follows (see also Figure 127):

A B C SCHEDULE OF ACTION
FOR COLITIS

A	B	C	D	E
St-21 37 39	Sp-15	B-20 27	K-13	L-7

(See Figure 127)

Supplementary
Procedures

1. *Coldpacks* on the belly nightly before bedtime. One hour per treatment.
2. *Dietary controls.*
   a. *Liberal fluid intake.*
   b. *Soft diet* (soups) with multiple meals, rather than a large evening meal.
   c. *Contraindications:*
      1. *All concentrated food mixtures*, with powdered milk, yeast, and proteins.
   d. *Vitamin B complex* and iron.

CONSTIPATION

Constipation is a static condition of the large intestine in which waste, standing still, not only leads to difficult defecation, or no defecation, but contributes to toxic waste in the body.

There are many strange ideas about bowel movements. Some people "go" normally two or three times a day in direct proportion

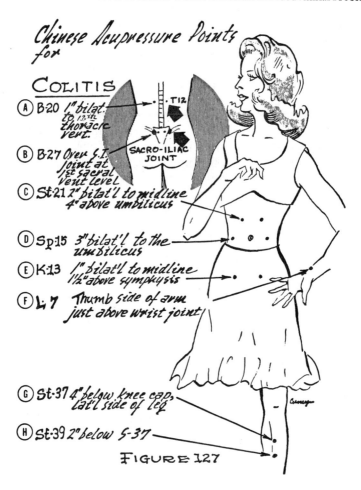

Chinese Acupressure Points for

COLITIS

(A) B-20 1" bilat. to 12th thoracic vert.

(B) B-27 Over S.I. joint at 1st sacral vert. level

(C) St-21 2" bilat'l to midline 4" above umbilicus

(D) Sp-15 3" bilat'l to the umbilicus

(E) K-13 1" bilat'l to midline 1½" above symphysis

(F) L-7 Thumb side of arm just above wrist joint

(G) St-37 4" below knee cap, lat'l side of leg

(H) St-39 2" below S-37

T-12

SACRO-ILIAC JOINT

FIGURE 127

to the amount of food they consume and the habits they have developed. Others may take two or three days before they defecate once. A static colon of this type is said to be "unstable" and has usually developed from the overuse of laxatives, purges, and even enemas. Quite often it may stem from failing to respond to the urge to evacuate when it comes, a lack of exercise, insufficient liquids throughout the day, or, an inadequate diet. There are many causes for constipation. Fatigue, drugs, malnutrition, and psychological problems are just a few.

How Carl Conquered His Constipation

Carl was a patient of mine. Living in his tense little world, he didn't have time to answer the "call of Nature." As a result, his "cesspool" backed up and he vomited at times. Part of the time he had severe belly pain. Sometimes he even passed blood when the stool finally came. He had no desire to eat, had a coated tongue, and was full of gas, and his abdomen was distended to the point that he couldn't even get his pants zippered together anymore. He was dizzy, had headaches, and suffered a slight fever. He also had a job that worried him to death, and the pressures brought to bear on him, the responsibilities, the headaches, were making him a nervous wreck. After using *Acupressure, U.S.A.* and showing him how he could treat himself in the future, I advised finding a new job. He did. No more constipation! It was as simple as that. Here are the key acupuncture points we used. See Figure 128.

A B C SCHEDULE OF ACTION
FOR CONSTIPATION

A	B	C	D	E	F	G	H
Li-6	St-36 36	Sp-15	B-25 33	K-1 16	H-5	GB-27 34	L-3

(See Figure 128)

Supplementary Procedures

1. *Physical therapy.*

   a. *Hotpacks* on back from seventh thoracic vertebra down to include the tail bone. One hour daily. Twice daily for one week if you have time for it.

   b. *Massage* the abdomen deeply but gently. Give special attention to the solar plexus area. Also relax all back muscles.

   c. *Salt water enema*, applied with a fountain syringe where bowels fail to react to the above treatment. (It is more than

Chinese Acupressure Points
for
CONSTIPATION

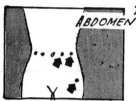
ABDOMEN

K·16 1"bilat'l to umbilicus

Sp 15 3" • •   •

GB·27 Anterior superior
iliac spine

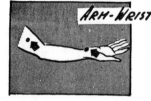
ARM-WRIST

H 5 Above wrist (little
finger side)

L 3 Midpoint on upper arm

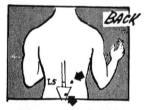
BACK

Li 6 Forearm lat'l side
above wrist

B·25 1½"bilat'l to 5th
lumbar vertebra

B 33 Over 3rd sacral vert

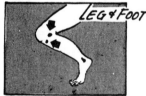
LEG & FOOT

GB·34 Lat'l side of knee
over head of fibula

St·36 1½" below knee cap
lat'l side

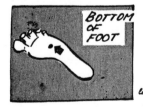
BOTTOM
OF
FOOT

K·1 Bottom of the foot,
behind 4th
metatarsal head

FIGURE 128

probable that the plug has to be loosened.) Solution: 1
tablespoonful per quart of water.

2. *Dietary controls.*

High residual foods eaten to excite peristalsis in bowel

wall. (Example—corn, cabbage, squash, cauliflower, potatoes, etc.)

   b. *Avoid all cathartics!* They contribute to the delinquency of a bowel and result in additional spasm.

   c. *Vitamin B complex with thiamine* added to diet.

3. *Habits.*

   a. *Go to the toilet* immediately on demand.

DIARRHEA

Diarrhea is that abnormally frequent discharge of fluid fecal matter that sometimes knows no apparent end.

In any language diarrhea comes out the same way, and no matter what the cause in the end it's not fun. Diarrhea may stem from fever diseases, acute enteritis, colitis, uremia, obstructive kidney problems, heart or liver diseases, food poisoning, psychic disturbances, intestinal parasites, defective chewing of food, etc. Going to a foreign land may do it.

Most diarrhea occurs in the summer. It may be the result of neglect, improper eating, impure water or milk, or a dozen other problems, including trips to Mexico. United States citizens, visiting in Mexico, are hard hit by what has been laughingly called *"Montezuma's Revenge"* or *"Tourista."* Of the many approaches used to treat this problem, I found *Acupressure, U.S.A.* the most practical.

To demonstrate how well it worked, let's take an experience aboard an airplane from Acapulco. Almost all the passengers aboard were wearing a lane to the back of the plane. My family started to show the same symptoms and signs, and I started treating acupuncture points designed to keep our bowels under control. What began with overindulgence in the hotels, change of environment, etc., was put under control. Those who took drugs for the matter kept on running to the toilet. Some even went to the hospital. My family went almost scot-free. The acupuncture points used are in the ABC Schedule on page 248.

Other than from travel in foreign lands, there are other reasons for diarrhea, and some of them are very serious. Where the problem is affecting you for the first time, check for obvious causes such as indigestible, green, or even overripe fruit. Food poisoning may be a possibility. Sudden weather changes are contributing factors. Fear and other emotions also play a role. But when the problem happens, use *Acupressure, U.S.A.* The cause doesn't matter in mild problems. The end results *do!* Here's how to do it.

A B C SCHEDULE OF ACTION
FOR DIARRHEA

A	B	C	D	E	F	G
St-21 44	Li-2 3	XM-2 (R side only)	Sp-3	H-6	B-21 65	K- 2 16

(See Figure 129)

**Supplementary
Procedures**

1. *Physical therapy.*
   a. *Coldpacks* immediately on the lower thoracic and upper lumbar area.
   b. *Massage* and thoroughly relax all neck and back muscles. Massage abdomen deeply but gently, with final emphasis on the solar plexus area.
2. *Dietary controls.*
   a. *Soft, bland diet.*
   b. *Vitamin B complex and iron.*
3. *Special acupuncture point technique as follows:*

Technique:

(a) *Pressure on the medulla oblongata area.* Place the third finger of each hand into the hollow at the base of your skull. Press. Hold. Repeat with rotation until all tenderness has receded.

(b) *Pressure on the umbilicus.* Insert all fingers of both hands into this area. Press. Hold for the five count. Release. Breathe deeply. Repeat for ten or more repetitions.

(c) *Palmar pressure on the abdomen.* Gently follow the course of the large intestine with regular on-and-off pressures. Start at the lower right of the abdomen up to the ribs; make a left turn across to the left side of the ribs; move down the left side of the abdomen, following the course of the descending colon, and over to the center.

(d) *Hip technique.* Check your hips. Note the painful area over the bony protuberance where the thigh bone makes a right angle turn to go into the joint. Locate each area of tenderness. Press each until the discomfort subsides.

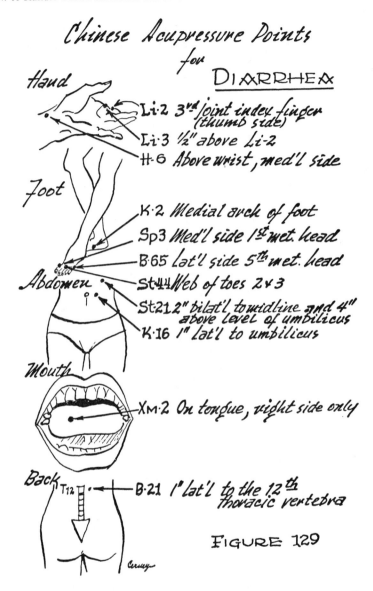

Chinese Acupressure Points for DIARRHEA

Hand
- Li·2 3rd joint index finger (thumb side)
- Li·3 ½" above Li·2
- H·6 Above wrist, med'l side

Foot
- K·2 Medial arch of foot
- Sp3 Med'l side 1st met. head
- B·65 Lat'l side 5th met. head
- St·44 Web of toes 2 x 3
- St·21 2" bilat'l to midline and 4" above level of umbilicus
- K·16 1" lat'l to umbilicus

Abdomen

Mouth
- Xm·2 On tongue, right side only

Back
- B·21 1" lat'l to the 12th thoracic vertebra

FIGURE 129

(e) *Low back and sacrum.* If you are in a seated position, just put your fists behind you. Lean back so that the knuckles are into the hollow on either side of your spinal column. Remain in this position a few minutes. Then place them lower down on the sacrum and repeat.

(f) *Armpit, arms, and scapula.* Check the armpit for nodules. If there are none, proceed to locate tenderness areas in the muscles from neck to shoulder. Locate all "ouch spots" and acupress. Put pressure on each side of the upper thoracic vertebrae because it is these important nerves that control many activities of the abdomen.

(g) *Web of first and second toes.* Liver meridian acupuncture point 3 is in the web of the great toe and its neighbor. Get your fingertip into the web. Investigate it for sore areas. Probe deep and you will locate a pinpoint of pain. This especially painful point is your key. Treat it. The moment the pain begins to ease, you can be assured that the abdominal organs with which it is associated will be in the same condition. In just this manner are all abdominal organs brought under control, or strengthened, and it's up to you to do the job. It's so convenient, so handy, just waiting to be used!

4. *Avoid all conditions that provoke diarrhea.*

GALL BLADDER PROBLEMS

NOTE: *Gall bladder problems are not usually home-style, self-help situations, but since acupuncture without needles is concerned with pain relief, here are emergency methods to use.*

Cholecystitis
(Acute Gall Bladder Emergency)

Just to the right of the solar plexus area, below the rib cage, a pain-sensitive area develops when the gall bladder begins to fill overly much and the thickened bile gives rise to pain and tenderness. If obstruction occurs, the bile dumps into the bloodstream and its yellow coloring matter appears in the skin. This problem is called "jaundice." The liver and gall bladder are directly related, and when anything affects the course of their normal action, certain reactions take place. These reactions are not locally confined.

For example, when the *Gall Bladder meridian* is getting interference, the person with the problem will notice that he has a bitter taste in his mouth. He will sigh frequently. His ribs and chest will ache. There will be pain at his temples, pain at the outer corner of each eye, and pain below the jaws. There will be swelling in front of the neck and swelling in the clavicular fossa, and in the armpits as well. The skin will perspire for no reason at all.

Traditional Chinese stated that the gall bladder was supposed to purify *Yang*. If the gall bladder is closed up for any reason, the *Yang* is encapsulated. It can't get loose into the body. The result is that a train of symptoms follow: insomnia, dizziness, vomiting, coated tongue, a feeling of sadness and melancholy. If there is too much *Yang*, then the symptoms change. Even the personality changes. Vision gets a little foggy, the ears don't hear as well, the ribs are painful, the pulse is fast, and a bitter taste comes up out of the stomach into the mouth. A person with this problem is headachy and nervous. He simply can't rest, can't sit down, can't lie down. His legs get weak, his chest feels full, his skin changes to a dusty hue.

People with an overactive gall bladder often have abdominal cramps, pain referred up between the shoulder blades and right arm. It may be referred down the back and into the right thigh. To handle this problem, use the following. Press the buttons. Nature does the rest. See Figure 130.

A B C SCHEDULE OF ACTION
FOR GALL BLADDER
PROBLEMS

A	B	C	D	E	F
GB-34 37 44	Liv-8	Tw-1	B-19	Gv-1	Check "Z" zones in foot (Fig. 23)

(See Figure 130)

Supplementary
Procedures

1. *Physical therapy.*

   a. *Icepack* on spine between the sixth and twelfth thoracic vertebrae.

   b. *Hotpacks* over the liver and gall bladder. Treat daily for a week. Alternate hot and cold for a week; thereafter, 15 minutes for each for one hour, at which time massage the back.

   c. *Massage back* in dorsal and lumbar region. Massage abdomen *gently* after the first three days. Give special attention to the liver area. It must be activated!

   d. *Cold water enema* where problem persists. Drink a lot of water as well.

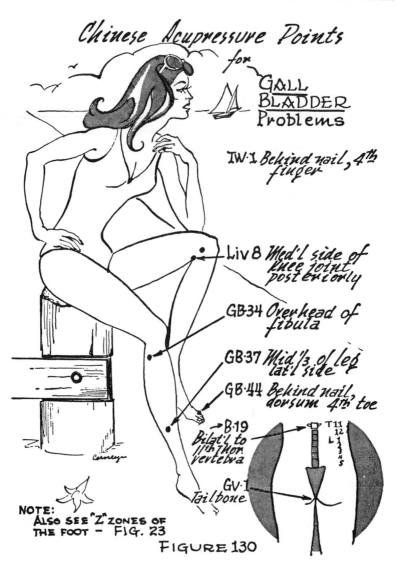

Chinese Acupressure Points

for

GALL
BLADDER
Problems

TW·1 *Behind nail, 4th finger*

Liv 8 *Med'l side of knee joint, posteriorly*

GB·34 *Overhead of fibula*

GB·37 *Mid 1/3 of leg lat'l side*

GB·44 *Behind nail, dorsum 4th toe*

→B·19 *Bilat'l to 11th Thor. vertebra*

GV·1 *Tailbone*

T 11
12
L 1
2
3
4
5

NOTE:
ALSO SEE "Z" ZONES OF
THE FOOT — FIG. 23

FIGURE 130

2. *Dietary controls.*

    a. DONT'S: *Avoid* all starches, fats, and sugars. *Avoid* peas, carrots, sweet vegetables, and sweet fruit. No egg yolks.

    b. DO'S: *Do* have fresh green vegetables. *Do* have fresh meat twice daily. *Do* have cereals that are *well cooked.*

GASTRITIS

Gastritis is inflammation of the stomach wall from any cause. Jock D. was a horse racing follower. He bet on everything and anything. He even bet on his health lasting forever, and then began to lose. That's when I saw him.

Jock is an older man who drinks coffee and booze non-stop. He smokes in between bites and in bed. He eats heavily of pastries and meat, and because his teeth are terrible, he simply swallows everything whole. When he came into my office his complaint was about "heartburn" and a scalding feeling in his throat. He said his appetite was good but that he had alternating constipation and diarrhea. Lately he'd been having headaches and dizziness.

But when he started throwing up after only a few drinks, that was it! He had to see Doc! He reported that he had lost weight and that after eating there was a funny fullness in his belly. He said he had a craving for highly seasoned and acid foods. I made all the necessary tests and examinations that proved out the diagnosis.

Gastritis! I told him what had to be done and he didn't like it. He would not get false teeth to help him chew. He would not change his diet or give up coffee, booze, or highly spiced foods or pastries. "What do you want me to do?" he growled, "stop living?". I shrugged and told him the choice was his and gave him a plan of action. He finally agreed to follow the ABC Schedule of Action laid out. Today Jock is back at the track again. His favorite spot is just to the right of the betting booths, and he'll give you hot tips anytime. The last hot tip he gave to me was a hayburner that dropped dead at the starter's gate. Age and hardening of the arteries had finally taken their toll ... on the horse.

A B C SCHEDULE OF ACTION
FOR GASTRITIS

A	B	C	D	E
St-21 36	B-61	K-12 20	Sp-1 16	See "Z" zones in foot (Fig. 23)

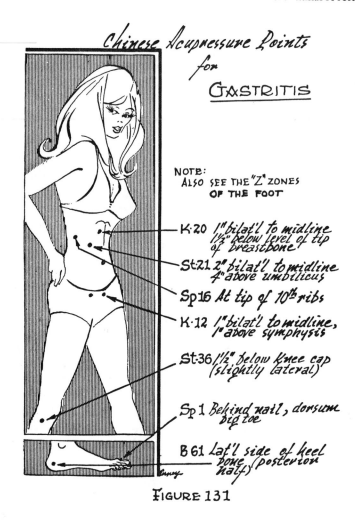

Chinese Acupressure Points
for
GASTRITIS

NOTE:
ALSO SEE THE "Z" ZONES
OF THE FOOT

K·20 *1" bilat'l to midline*
1½" below level of tip
of breastbone

St·21 *2" bilat'l to midline*
4" above umbilicus

Sp 16 *At tip of 10th ribs*

K·12 *1" bilat'l to midline,*
1" above symphysis

St·36 *1½" below knee cap*
(slightly lateral)

Sp 1 *Behind nail, dorsum*
big toe

B 61 *Lat'l side of heel*
bone (posterior
half)

FIGURE 131

Supplementary
Procedures

    1. *Physical therapy.*
        a. *Icepack* on abdomen. Time: one hour.
        b. *Additional pressure techniques.*

Technique:

    (a) *Mid-thoracic pressure.* There are two methods for handling this problem. One is to have a buddy applying his thumbs on your back at the sides of each thoracic vertebra. Starting at the top, move down. This is best done by lying face-down on a table or sofa. Your buddy is leaning forward and over you, his full weight bearing down on his thumbs. He must hold each position for the five count. Release. When he comes to a particular point of pain, tell him so. At this point, compress the area at least five times or until the point of pain is gone. If pain persists, it indicates chronicity in the gastric organ, so persist.

The second method for accomplishing this same procedure is through the use of golf balls. Place them on the hard floor. Lie back on them. Press. Hold. Repeat downwardly to include each thoracic nerve.

(b) *Fingertip pressure on the solar plexus.* Lie on your back. Place the fingertips of both hands in your solar plexus. Hold for the five count. Breathe deeply. Release. Repeat process for five minutes. Place the icepack on your belly and go to sleep.

HEMORRHOIDS
AND OTHER
RECTAL PROBLEMS

Hemorrhoids are varicosed or dilated blood vessels in or around the anus. Sooner or later, all of us—for one reason or another—have a rectal disorder. The area may fissure, have a cyst or abscess, fistula, itch, hemorrhoids or proctitis may develop, etc.—all pesky involvements that are not just embarrassing, but contribute to a great deal of pain and discomfort—and *Acupressure, U.S.A.* becomes a good modality to use.

To determine the extent or chronicity of your rectal problem, probe the reflex area just behind and above the inner ankle bone. In size, this zone of tenderness may range from pinpoint hurt to an area an inch wide and 3 inches long between the tibia and the Achilles tendon. Size and tenderness are directly proportional to the duration and complications of the rectal problem causing it.

Trigger points for rectal hemorrhoids may be found on either side of the Achilles tendon. Another trigger point may be noted at the very tip of the tail bone. You have only to use these acupuncture points to your advantage.

A Showgirl Demonstrates
Her End Product

Sue Ann was one rectal patient I didn't mind looking at. She was a curvaceous showgirl. Along with her beautiful figure and brains, she also had *pruritus ani.* What's pruritus ani? The itch! It's around the rectum. Whenever there is warmth and moisture, or hemorrhoids, this itching becomes almost unbearable. Worse at night. Especially worse when sweating. At first I suspected hemorrhoids in Ann's case, but that didn't check out. After exhausting the possible causes, I began to realize that this was an unusually healthy young woman.

But why the red mass of itching that was apparently making her frantic? She'd been to clinics in various cities with no results. The scratch-itch cycle was "driving her mad" by her own confession. When I finally determined the cause and started pressing the vital acupuncture points, it all stopped.

What caused her problem? *Monilia! Monilia* is a fungus found normally in the vagina. After urinating, she'd wipe herself backwardly toward the anus. The parasites invaded 'their new habitat and simply set up housekeeping. The area was ideal for their proliferation.

I demonstrated how to use *Acupressure, U.S.A.* as follows, and added some rules and regulations on anal hygiene. This included low residual diet for soft bowel movements and cleansing the anus with water-moistened pledgets of cotton.

A B C SCHEDULE OF ACTION
FOR MOST RECTAL PROBLEMS

A	B	C	D	E	F	G*	H
L-7	Sp-1 20 8	Si-5	B-18 65	K-8	GB-39	P-4 8	GV-1

*Also see "Z" zones of the foot for hemorrhoids (Figure 23).

Weeks later, I received a letter from Sue Ann. She was in a Broadway tune show. She addressed me in a naval manner:

Dear Rear Admiral:

There are not enough words to tell you how thankful I am for relieving my rectal problem. Every day now I treat those Oriental pressure points as you prescribed and stick to the rules of proper hygiene, and there hasn't been a re-occurrence since I last saw you. I

Chinese Acupressure Points
for
HEMORRHOIDS

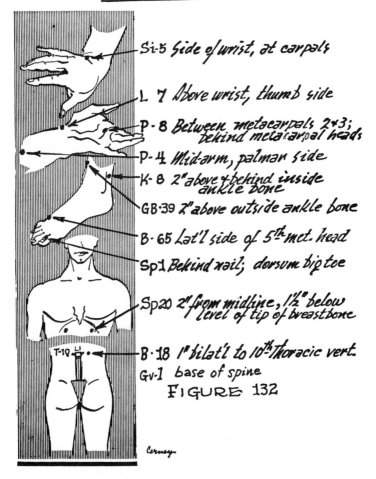

Si-5 *Side of wrist, at carpals*

L·7 *Above wrist, thumb side*

P·8 *Between metacarpals 2 & 3; behind metacarpal heads*

P·4 *Mid-arm, palmar side*

K·8 *2" above & behind inside ankle bone*

GB·39 *2" above outside ankle bone*

B·65 *Lat'l side of 5th met. head*

Sp·1 *Behind nail; dorsum big toe*

Sp·20 *2" from midline, 1½" below level of tip of breastbone*

B·18 *1" bilat'l to 10th Thoracic vert.*

Gv·1 *base of spine*

FIGURE 132

thought I was through with show biz, but now I'm doing better than ever. With your help, the amazing thing about this Chinese kind of treatment for rectal problems is that I was bound to improve in the end.

Sue Ann

Supplementary
Procedures

   1. *Physical therapy.*
      a. *Deep massage* all tissues of the sacral and lumbar area.
      b. *Avoid all violent forms of exercise.* This includes heavy lifting and long walks as well as horseback riding.
      c. *Coldpack* on sacrum and rectal area.
   2. *Dietary control.*
      a. *Don't* eat highly seasoned food.
      b. *Don't* drink alcoholic beverages or coffee or cola drinks.
      c. *Do* eat easily digested foods. Drink lots of water.
   3. *Hygiene.*
      a. Wash anus with water after each bowel movement. *Don't* use colored tissues (the dye in the paper is an inflammatory agent).
      b. Evacuate bowels daily.

HERNIA

Hernia is any break in the abdominal wall permitting the external projection of some part of the abdominal contents.

Acupuncture is admittedly of lesser value where musculature is ripped or torn and the bowels protrude. However, for relief of discomfort and for lesser hernias, acupuncture *can* be of value. It's a method of choice, and for this purpose the Chinese advocate the following:

A B C SCHEDULE OF ACTION
FOR HERNIA

A	B	C	D
St-27 30 33	Sp-5 12	B-29 55	K-14

(See Figure 133)

INDIGESTION

Indigestion, also called *dyspepsia*, is a symptom of imperfect digestion from one or more causes.

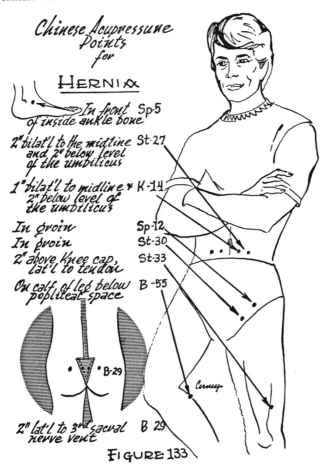

Chinese Acupressure Points for

HERNIA

In front of inside ankle bone — Sp-5

2" bilat'l to the midline and 2" below level of the umbilicus — St-27

1" bilat'l to midline & 2" below level of the umbilicus — K-14

In groin — Sp-12

In groin — St-30

2" above knee cap, lat'l to tendon — St-33

On calf of leg below popliteal space — B-55

• B-29

2" lat'l to 3rd sacral nerve vent — B 29

FIGURE 133

People have died from "acute indigestion" when the use of acupuncture points would have kept them alive. Anyone having this problem will have "heartburn," nausea, pain in the upper abdomen, distension of the abdomen because of gas, and all of this occurring during or immediately after eating.

A Computer Operator Defeats Indigestion

Frances J. is an IBM operator. Ten years ago, she started developing a feeling of faintness, dizziness, and sometimes headaches. Then came the regurgitation of her stomach contents, and "burning" or "heartburn" traveling up her esophagus. Excessive gastric acidity came up in a burning mess. Accumulated gas exploded both ways. Acupuncture pressure techniques proved highly efficacious for her problem. But *the real key to her problem was the set of trigger points over her left breast* all of which were exquisitely tender. The moment they were treated, with rotary pressure, the "attack of indigestion" stopped! Here are the controls I used.

A B C SCHEDULE OF ACTION
FOR INDIGESTION

A	B	C	D	E	F
St-16	Li-8 10	Sp-2 7 20	B-66	K-14 24	"Z" zones of the foot (Fig. 23)

Supplementary Procedures

1. *Physical therapy.*

   a. *Heatpacks* applied over vagus nerve on the sides of the neck and over the solar plexus.

   b. *Coldpacks* simultaneously over the thoracic vertebrae for at least 30 minutes once daily.

   c. *Massage* all muscles of the back and abdomen gently but firmly till loose.

   d. *Daily cold sponge bath* followed by a brisk rough towel rubdown.

2. *Dietary controls.*

   a. *Balanced diet* to be maintained at all times. Eat slowly. Spend at least three quarters of an hour eating each meal. Chew thoroughly without haste!

   b. *Control circumstance and environment* by avoiding everything and anything unpleasant.

   c. *Contraindications:*

   (1) Gossip, anger, sarcasm, and everything else where you are emotionally involved. Avoid conflict. Walk away.

   (2) Going without rest detracts from digestion. Rest daily before and after each meal. Your biggest responsibility is maintaining your personal health. Do it with planned

action because all such factors are intimately tied into the acupuncture points you use.

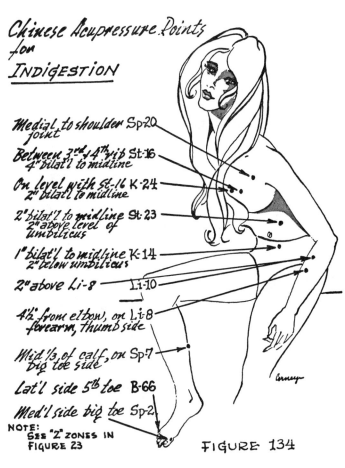

Chinese Acupressure Points
for
INDIGESTION

Medial to shoulder Sp-20
   joint

Between 3rd & 4th rib St-16
   4" bilat'l to midline

On level with St-16 K-24
   2" bilat'l to midline

2" bilat'l to midline St-23
   2" above level of
   umbilicus

1" bilat'l to midline K-14
   2" below umbilicus

2" above Li-8   Li-10

4½" from elbow, on Li-8
   forearm, thumb side

Mid ⅓ of calf, on Sp-7
   big toe side

Lat'l side 5th toe B-66

Med'l side big toe Sp-2

NOTE:
   SEE "Z" ZONES IN
   FIGURE 23

FIGURE 134

NAUSEA

Nausea is that feeling of distress accompanied by the desire to vomit.

Nausea, as a symptom, has varied causes and is closely associated with vomiting. Nausea occurring *after* a headache may be due to an eye problem or migraine. Morning nausea may be due to gastritis, kidney problems, or even pregnancy. It may even be a symptom of jaundice, with the liver and gall bladder involved. It may be the result of a cardiac complication. Nausea may be present in car, air, or sea sickness. It may be due to "nerves," hysteria, or the sight or smell of something obnoxious. Nausea may be present without vomiting. But in either case, with or without, here is the Oriental approach.

A B C SCHEDULE OF ACTION
FOR NAUSEA

A	B	C	D	E	F	G
L-3	H-1	B-41	St-21	P-4	GB-14	Gv-16

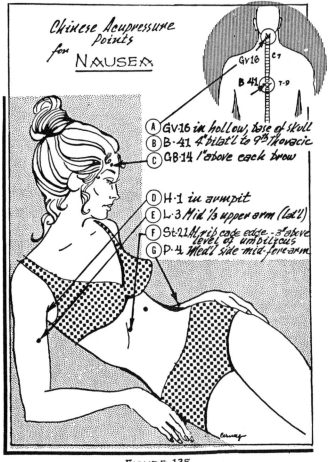

FIGURE 135

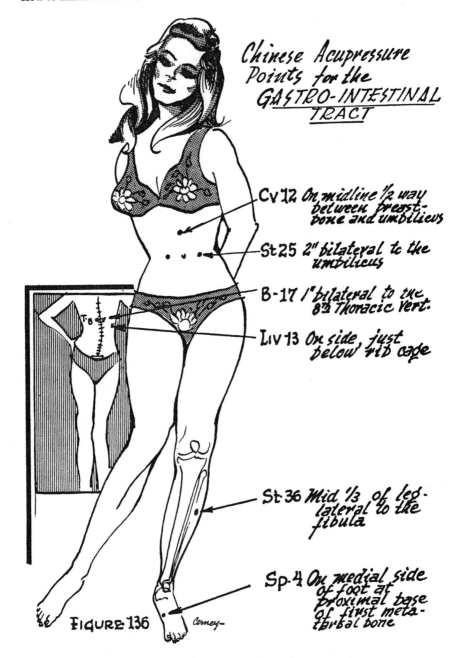

Chinese Acupressure Points for the GASTRO-INTESTINAL TRACT

Cv 12 On midline ½ way between breast-bone and umbilicus

St 25 2" bilateral to the umbilicus

B-17 1" bilateral to the 8th Thoracic Vert.

Liv 13 On side, just below rib cage

St 36 Mid ⅓ of leg - lateral to the fibula

Sp. 4 On medial side of foot at proximal base of first meta-tarsal bone

FIGURE 136

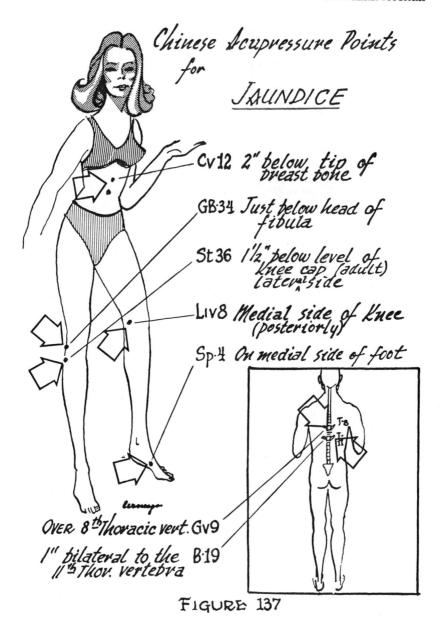

Chinese Acupressure Points
for
JAUNDICE

Cv 12   2" below tip of breast bone

GB·34   Just below head of fibula

St 36   1½" below level of knee cap (adult) lateral side

Liv 8   Medial side of knee (posteriorly)

Sp·4   On medial side of foot

OVER 8th Thoracic vert. Gv 9

1" bilateral to the 11th Thov. vertebra   B·19

FIGURE 137

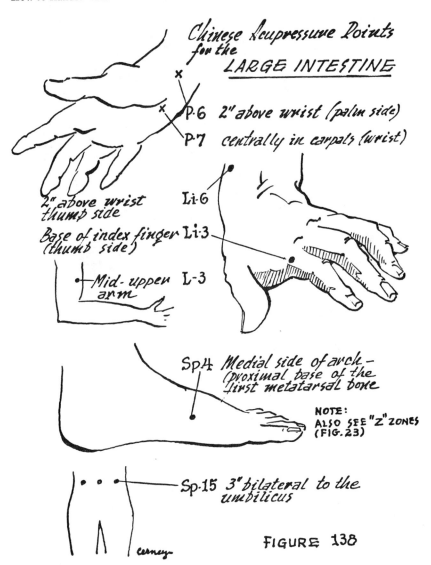

Chinese Acupressure Points
for the
LARGE INTESTINE

P·6 2" above wrist (palm side)

P·7 centrally in carpals (wrist)

2" above wrist
thumb side   Li·6

Base of index finger Li·3
(thumb side)

Mid·upper   L·3
arm

Sp4 Medial side of arch —
(proximal base of the
first metatarsal bone

NOTE:
ALSO SEE "Z" ZONES
(FIG. 23)

Sp·15 3" bilateral to the
umbilicus

FIGURE 138

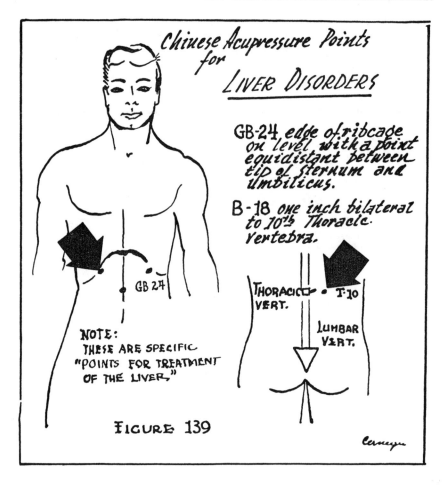

Chinese Acupressure Points for LIVER DISORDERS

GB-24 edge of ribcage on level with a point equidistant between tip of sternum and umbilicus.

B-18 one inch bilateral to 10th Thoracic Vertebra.

NOTE: THESE ARE SPECIFIC "POINTS FOR TREATMENT OF THE LIVER."

FIGURE 139

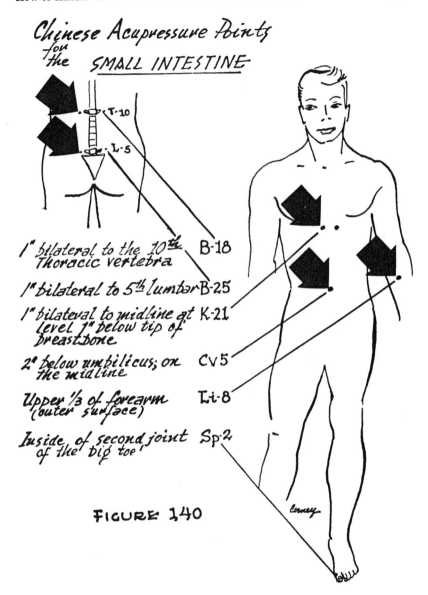

Chinese Acupressure Points
for
the SMALL INTESTINE

1" bilateral to the 10th Thoracic vertebra B-18

1" bilateral to 5th lumbar B-25

1" bilateral to midline at K-21 level 1" below tip of breastbone

2" below umbilicus; on CV5 the midline

Upper 1/3 of forearm Li-8 (outer surface)

Inside of second joint Sp-2 of the big toe

FIGURE 140

Supplementary
Procedures

   1. *Physical therapy.*
      a. *Icepack* at base of skull and one over the solar plexus
   area. Treatment time, 30 minutes.
      b. *Massage* muscles of back, with special attention to the
   sore areas alongside the spinal column.

BONUS THERAPIES
FOR THE GASTRO-INTESTINAL SYSTEM
AND ABDOMINAL ORGANS

   How-to-do-it acupuncture points to use and schedules to follow
will give you a new lease on life.
   See Figures 136-140 on:

   a. *General gastro-intestinal care.*
   b. *Jaundice.*
   c. *Large intestine.*
   d. *Liver disorders.*
   e. *Small intestine.*

HOW TO HANDLE PELVIS AND HIP AILMENTS

The Pelvis . . . and
How Pain Is Referred

   Sexual organs, in the pelvis, are the victims of inflammation,
and even displacement at times. The pregnant uterus or painful
menstruation (dysmenorrhea), for example, may each express discomfort in a different way. Pains originating in a pelvic lesion may
reflexly re-distribute to the mammary glands, to the back of the
head, to the front of the thigh, or even to the lateral and back side of
the hip. When ovaries are diseased, pain may be referred to the wrist
or even to the heel of the foot. In ailments of the uterus, there may
be pain reflexly projected to the hands.
   In the male, when the prostate is involved, he may have pain
referred to the ankle or into the soles of his feet. Involvement of the
testicles may cause pain beneath the sacrum and tail bone. A
testicular varicocele (a varicose vein on the gonad) may contribute to

pain in the groin. Cystitis may contribute to pubic pain. Hernial pain may refer itself to the knee as does a "sick hip." Where there are hemorrhoids in the rectum, the sacrum and coccyx become painful at times.

In the above examples, you see an amazing story of how pain is referred from one point to another, and this is a key story in acupuncture.

Each of these pains follows nerve patterns and meridians. In the following illustration, you will see how inflammation and disease in one body part pop up somewhere else, and where they surface, a "trigger point" is accentuated. The trigger point may also be very near. For example the trigger point for hemorrhoids is just under the tip of the coccyx. These are human electronic buttons . . . pressure zones . . . waiting for your fingertips to help you achieve peace of body and mind!

Brief, At-a-Glance Techniques for *PELVIS and HIP*

Procedure: Check your symptoms. Find the acupuncture point . . . acupress!

A B C SCHEDULE OF ACTION

SYMPTOMS	ACUPUNCTURE POINTS TO USE				
	A	B	C	D	E
Arthritis in hip (pain)	Li-18	B-27, 28	GB-26 29, 30	St-31	St-40 41
Pain in hip	Li-18				
Sacro-iliitis	B-28	B-29			
Sciatica	B-26, 28	B-48, 49	B-50	Gv-3	
Stiffness and pain	GB-30	GB-34			

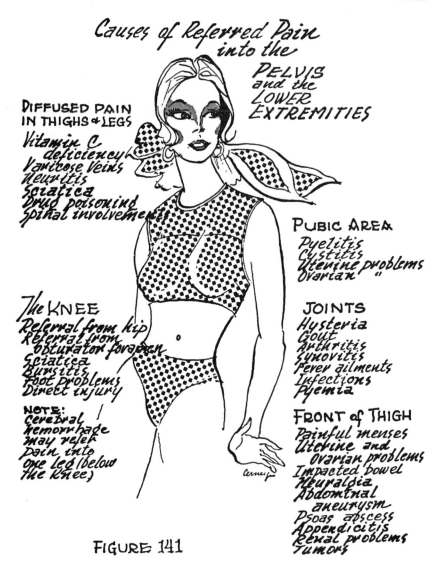

Causes of Referred Pain into the PELVIS and the LOWER EXTREMITIES

DIFFUSED PAIN IN THIGHS & LEGS
Vitamin C deficiency
Varicose Veins
Neuritis
Sciatica
Drug poisoning
Spinal involvements

The KNEE
Referral from hip
Referral from obturator foramen
Sciatica
Bursitis
Foot problems
Direct injury

NOTE:
Cerebral hemorrhage may refer pain into one leg (below the knee)

PUBIC AREA
Pyelitis
Cystitis
Uterine problems
Ovarian "

JOINTS
Hysteria
Gout
Arthritis
Synovitis
Fever ailments
Infections
Pyemia

FRONT of THIGH
Painful menses
Uterine and Ovarian problems
Impacted bowel
Neuralgia
Abdominal aneurysm
Psoas abscess
Appendicitis
Renal problems
Tumors

FIGURE 141

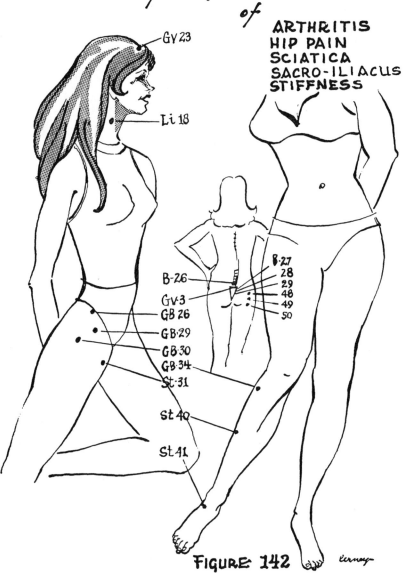

MASTER PLAN for Acupressure Treatment of

**ARTHRITIS
HIP PAIN
SCIATICA
SACRO-ILIACUS
STIFFNESS**

GV 23

Li 18

B-26
GV-3
GB 26
GB-29
GB-30
GB-34
St-31

St 40

St 41

B-27
28
29
48
49
50

FIGURE 142

HOW TO HANDLE
AILMENTS OF LEGS AND FEET

10

This chapter is unique in that it gives you illustrations and ABC's-of-Action in abbreviated form. The lower extremity is designated by anatomical segments to give you a more clear emphasis of the "where" of the treatment as well as of the discomfort or pain; viz: *buttock, thigh, knee, lower leg, ankle,* and *foot.*

Self-help procedures for each part are ready for you at a glance. Simply find the key acupuncture points on the illustration. Locate them on yourself. Probe. Locate the tenderness. Mark. Each will be identified by pinpoint pain. Sometimes an area of painful swelling may accompany it. Merely press these "magic buttons" as prescribed earlier. Nature will do the rest.

THREE METHODS FOR
CONQUERING PAIN AND RESTORING HEALTH
IN THE LOWER EXTREMITIES

Method 1: *Supplementary Physical Therapy*

To enhance the speed of acupuncture or acupressure procedures on the extremities, the nerve roots at the spinal column may be sedated or inspired by the use of cold or hot applications. Where the lower extremities are involved, apply a hotpack on the lower thoracic and lumbar areas. Time: 15 minutes. Follow with an icepack for 30 minutes. Treat twice daily. Follow with a thorough massage of the muscles of the buttocks and low back. Go one step further with your physical therapy procedure. Use an ice cube on the acupuncture points. Be methodical about it. Be precise. Be certain.

Method 2: *"Trigger Point" Therapy*

Trigger points may be of further aid to you in your conquest over discomfort and pain. The illustration that follows (Figure 143) demonstrates exactly where to control given parts of the lower extremities with the unique "trigger point" pressure. These triggers are vital to personal care and often serve when nothing else is available. Each trigger is notable in that it is accompanied by an acupuncture point in the same area. Each trigger-point-control area controls a defined segment of the anatomy within the range of its own major nerve segments. In using these triggers, you not only utilize the accompanying acupuncture point and the autonomic nervous system, but major mainline nerves as well. Study the illustration. If you have a pain in a given area of the extremity, locate it on the chart. Then locate it on yourself. Find the key! Press!

Method 3: *"Z" Zones . . . Health Control on the Foot That Can Change the Course of Your Life*

In treating the human body through pressure points—and in utilizing techniques of the traditional past—my Americanization of Oriental acupuncture makes it as American as Chinese *chop suey*. The Chinese ingredients are all there. We've just changed the recipe and added a personal touch. The Chinese indicate that there is only one acupuncture point on the bottom of the foot (Kidney 1), but we find a lot more, and each is a switchboard for reflex nerve control. With this in mind, I want to add to lower extremity care the dynamic power of the "Z" ZONES . . . reflex zones found on the bottom of the foot. (See Figure 23.)

I call them "Z" zones because they mark given zones on each foot. They too are triggers in reflexology and are associated with the autonomic nervous system, as well as the Chinese meridians that start on the dorsum of the foot. They are totally related with the mainline nervous system. Where these three methods are used to supplement the procedures of *acupuncture without needles*, you assure yourself of faster recovery. Combine these three methods in helping yourself to health. Don't expect fantastic cures immediately. Don't look for immediate miracles. But when they happen, be glad. In the meantime, keep working for your miracle by using fingertip controls on Nature. At your very fingertips *is* health, and if you would change the course of your life, it's up to you to use these methods efficaciously.

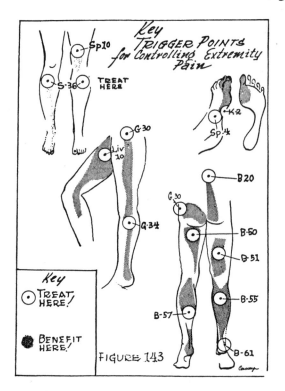

FIGURE 143

Please be reminded—in your care of the lower extremities—that *Acupressure, U.S.A.*, as a manual procedure, is a combination of methods that have been used behind the Bamboo Curtain for at least 50 centuries. Compressing trigger points on nerves and Chinese meridians is like pressing an electric light switch. Press the right button and a physiological phenomenon takes place! Use the magic of *your* physiological buttons. Here now are the anatomical segments. Each is accompanied by illustrations and an ABC Schedule of Action. Study those "Z" zones. Add them to the other procedures, and you will get the results you desire.

BUTTOCKS

**Farmer's Painful Accident
Conquered via Acupressure**

The buttocks, formed by the rounded mass of gluteal muscles, are a landing platform subject to various kinds of injury and pain. Many of the pains in the gluteals are referred pains. They stem from another source. In the general treatment of the buttocks and loins, the following illustrations show you how-to-do-it.

Cory F. is a farmer. While Spring plowing, his tractor hit a buried rock and he was bounced off the seat and landed on his rear. At the time, he didn't think anything about it. Then he started having pain in his low back and gluteals. The pain went all the way down to the knee after awhile, and that's when I saw him. His bottom was so tender he had to do everything standing up. How his buttock problem was conquered is illustrated in Figure 144. Along with the three methods described earlier, take advantage of those acupuncture points! They're there with a purpose!

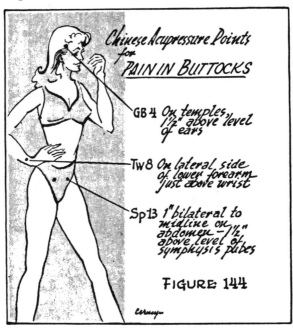

Chinese Acupressure Points for PAIN IN BUTTOCKS

GB 4 On temples, 1½" above level of ears

Tw 8 On lateral side of lower forearm just above wrist

Sp 13 1" bilateral to midline on abdomen — 1½" above level of symphysis pubes

FIGURE 144

A Stenographer Returns to Work After a Long Leave of Absence and Gross Pain

Judy H. is a stenographer. She sits all day pounding away at a typewriter. She wraps her feet around the legs of the chair and perches from cheek to cheek to relieve her bottom. After 15 years of this, pain hit her in the buttocks. It got progressively worse. She went to the hospital. No relief. There was no history of similar problems, but there was a history of hemorrhoids, white vaginal discharge, painful menstruation, and "weak" kidneys. She was always weary and out-of-sorts. But when treatment began on her *Bladder meridian*, all this changed. She said, "It's like magic! All my aches and pains are gone! It's a pleasure going back to work." And it was a pleasure for me too, because her high blood pressure went down. The ABC's of acupuncture points used are in Figure 144.

THIGHS

A Child's Agony Is Conquered via Acupressure, U.S.A.

Pain in the thighs was developed by a little lady we'll call Lorna. Most of the pain centered on the inner side of her thighs. It started first around the vulva and became progressively worse in agony until this seven-year-old was crying day and night. Drugs seemed valueless and ineffective. There was no redness, no swelling, just pain. Her mother was frantic. She reported that Lorna would wake up screaming; when she finally would go to sleep, she dreamed of ghosts; there were spasms in Lorna's feet; she had headaches; and her face was swollen. The child was in a constant state of agitation until office treatment and home treatment with *Acupressure, U.S.A.* began. With emphasis on *Spleen meridian* acupuncture point 5, came a little miracle. Lorna's pain stopped! She returned to school. The key acupuncture points that conquered this problem are in the following illustrations (Figures 145 and 146.)

PAINS IN THE KNEES

A Housewife's "Arthritis" Is Cured

Sarah C. complained of redness, swelling, and pain in her knees. On first thought it appeared to be arthritis, the way she self-diagnosed it. She also admitted to pain along the shaft of the big lower leg bone and swelling of her thighs. She said that sometimes her abdominal muscles went into spasm, and sometimes the same thing happened to her jaw muscles. When she indicated that her second

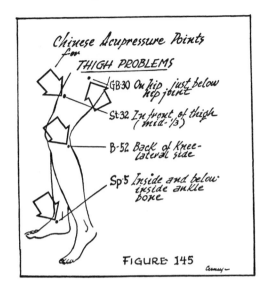

Chinese Acupressure Points
for
THIGH PROBLEMS

GB-30 On hip, just below
hip joint

St-32 In front of thigh
(mid-⅓)

B-52 Back of knee-
lateral side

Sp-5 Inside and below
inside ankle
bone

FIGURE 145

Chinese Acupressure Points

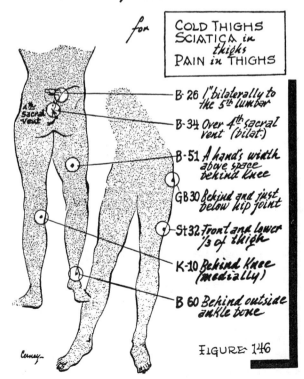

for

COLD THIGHS
SCIATICA in
thighs
PAIN in THIGHS

B-26 1" bilaterally to
the 5th lumbar

B-34 Over 4th sacral
vent (bilat.)

B-51 A hand's width
above space
behind knee

GB-30 Behind and just
below hip joint

St-32 Front and lower
⅓ of thigh

K-10 Behind knee
(medially)

B-60 Behind outside
ankle bone

FIGURE 146

and third toes went into spasm as well, I knew that the *Stomach meridian* and its muscle branches were involved. The Orientals have long known of this problem and have used the acupuncture points of the *Stomach meridian* and *Bladder meridian* to treat it. In Sarah C.'s case, treatment proved eminently successful. In her case, it didn't matter whether it was pseudo-arthritis or the real thing—the hurt was the same. So was the treatment. And here are the acupuncture points I used. They will help you too.

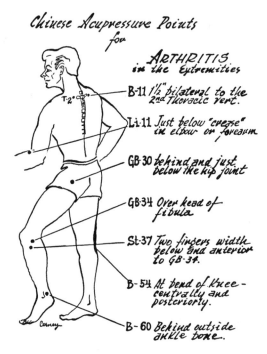

Chinese Acupressure Points
for
ARTHRITIS
in the Extremities

B-11 1½" bilateral to the 2nd Thoracic vert.

Li-11 Just below "crease" in elbow on forearm

GB-30 behind and just below the hip joint

GB-34 Over head of fibula

St-37 Two fingers width below and anterior to GB-34.

B-54 At bend of knee—centrally and posteriorly.

B-60 Behind outside ankle bone.

FIGURE 147

Bending or Flexing the Knee with Difficulty (Stiff Knee)

Comeback of Key
Gymnast Is Hastened

A stiff knee is not unique to any one age group, ·although it appears more often in the aged as joint changes take place. More often than not, the problem is *not* the knee joint itself but rather in the soft tissues around it. These are the muscles, fascia, ligaments, etc. that control the integrity of that knee joint and make the leg operate. For example when star gymnast Kate J. lost her grip on the parallel bars, and twisted her leg as she fell, her knee was quick to react to injury. X-ray film revealed nothing. Palpation of the soft tissues around the joint, the muscles, and tendons revealed her "ouch spots." All of them were in revolt from being tortured by the fall. *Acupressure, U.S.A.* was begun immediately. She healed fast and competed in the State Tournament to become All-State Women's Gymnast.

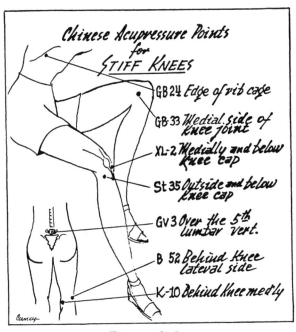

Chinese Acupressure Points for STIFF KNEES

GB24 *Edge of rib cage*
GB33 *Medial side of knee joint*
XL-2 *Medially and below knee cap*
St35 *Outside and below knee cap*
GV3 *Over the 5th lumbar vert.*
B 52 *Behind knee lateral side*
K-10 *Behind knee med'ly*

FIGURE 148

*Bone Diseases
Involving the Knee*

Football Star Recuperates from Bone Disease

High school football player Jackie M. had Osgood-Schlatter's disease, which is a problem of young people. The bump of bone to which the knee cap attaches, by way of a tendon, pulls away. Usually a blow starts it off. Symptoms are pain, swelling, and tenderness as the bone disorganizes locally. In Jackie's case, the surgeon did his bit and the physiotherapy department at the hospital did its bit. I did my bit and was somewhat chagrined at my ineffectiveness until Oriental acupuncture points were put to use. The key to all bone diseases is *Bladder meridian* acupuncture point 11, so I used it. Within a month, the bone was reorganized. Local tenderness was gone. The patellar tendon was in a fixed position. I never saw anything heal so fast, and after 25 years working with athletic injuries, this was a phenomenon to behold.

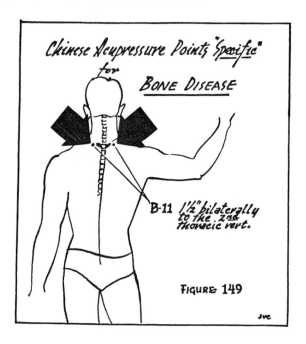

Chinese Acupressure Points "Specific" for BONE DISEASE

B-11 1½" bilaterally to the 2nd thoracic vert.

FIGURE 149

Cold Sensation
in the Knees

Mrs. N. and her icy-cold knees created some laughs with the other physicians who had attended her, and she stopped going. When she couldn't stand it any longer, she called me. She also complained of heartburn, vomiting, and hiccoughing. She said any pressure on her abdomen made her feel good, but she just couldn't go on living if that ice in her knees continued. Since these were all the symptoms of the insufficiency of the *Stomach meridian*, the necessary acupuncture points were used. (See Figure 150). She recuperated and came out of her negative personality complex also. The last time she was in for her check-up treatment, she was friendly, charming, personable, and said she had just joined the Women's League!

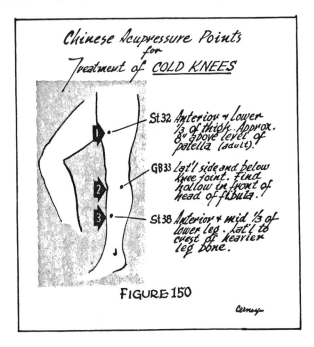

Chinese Acupressure Points
for
Treatment of COLD KNEES

St.32 Anterior + lower ⅓ of thigh. Approx. 8" above level of patella (adult).

GB33 lat'l side and below knee joint. Find hollow in front of head of fibula.

St.38 Anterior + mid ⅓ of lower leg. Lat'l to crest of heavier leg bone.

FIGURE 150

Numbness
in the Knees

See Figure 151 for treatment of numbness in the knees.

If you have numbness in your knees and your second and third toes are painful, it's possible your *Stomach meridian* is kicking up. The acupuncture points to use are shown in Figure 151.

Pain
in the Knees

The knees are often a referral point for pain from other body parts. As a shallow and rather inadequate flat joint, it presents a highly sensitive area for breeding hurt. Acupressure points which follow (see Figure 152) are vital in relieving pain from referred sources.

Swelling
in the Knees

In addition to the usual systemic causes for swelling in the

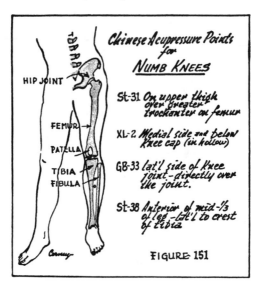

Chinese Acupressure Points
for
NUMB KNEES

HIP JOINT

FEMUR →
PATELLA
TIBIA
FIBULA

St-31 On upper thigh over greater trochanter on femur

XL-2 Medial side and below knee cap (in hollow)

GB-33 Lat'l side of knee joint—directly over the joint.

St-38 Anterior of mid-⅓ of leg—Lat'l to crest of tibia

FIGURE 151

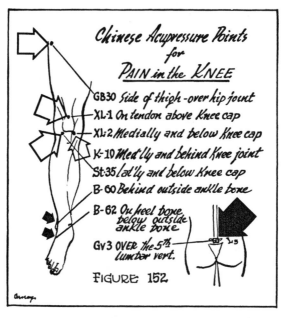

Chinese Acupressure Points
for
PAIN in the KNEE

GB30 Side of thigh—over hip joint
XL-1 On tendon above knee cap
XL-2 Medially and below knee cap
K-10 Med'lly and behind knee joint
St-35 Lat'ly and below knee cap
B-60 Behind outside ankle bone
B-62 On heel bone below outside ankle bone.
Gv3 OVER the 5th lumbar vert.

FIGURE 152

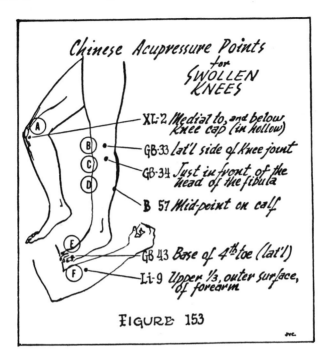

Chinese Acupressure Points for SWOLLEN KNEES

XL-2 *Medial to, and below knee cap (in hollow)*

GB-33 *lat'l side of knee joint*

GB-34 *Just in front of the head of the fibula*

B 57 *Mid-point on calf*

GB 43 *Base of 4th toe (lat'l)*

Li-9 *Upper ⅓, outer surface, of forearm*

FIGURE 153

extremities, the environment plays a role. In older folks, swelling in the knees may occur with every weather change. Coldness and wetness cause an immediate effect. To neutralize this problem, use the acupressure points in Figure 153.

LOWER LEG

How Acupressure Helped an Old Lady's Leg Ulcer

I showed an anxious patient with an aggravated case of leg ulcers how to use acupressure for it. In only two months, the leg ulcer was healed! Here she had had this open running sore for over 30 years! The great clinics had failed in healing it, yet *Acupressure, U.S.A.* healed it in two months! The "how to" lies in Figure 154.

Brief, At-a-Glance Techniques for *LEG PROBLEMS*

Procedure: Check your symptoms. Find the acupuncture points and acupress! (See Figure 154 for pressure locations.)

A B C SCHEDULE OF ACTION

SYMPTOMS   ACUPUNCTURE POINTS TO USE

	A	B	C	D	E
Can't raise leg	St-37	B-59			
Cold Feeling	St-23	St-33	K-1	K-6	Sp-2
Collapse	B-10				
Muscle cramps *medial side* of leg *lateral*	B-28, 29 Sp-9	B-50, 52	B-53, 55	B-59, 61	K-9
Not able to walk	Sp-7				
Pain	B-28		K-2		
Swelling	S-32	S-37			
Weakness in legs	XL-1	Sp-27, 36 73	Sp-9 14	B-25 28, 29 58, 61	K-9
Weariness	K-3	GB-34			

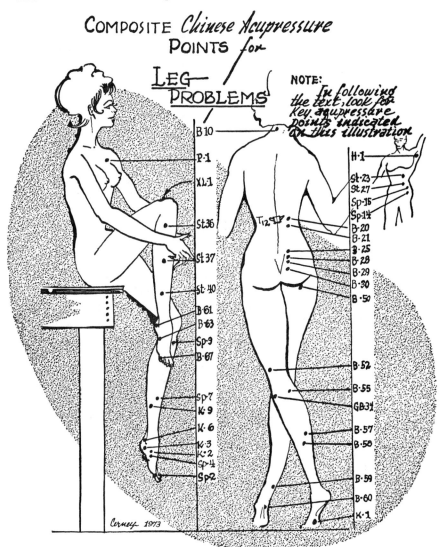

FIGURE 154

THE ANKLE

As a fairly secure and well-engineered joint, the ankle is not subject to a lot of problems. The more common problem is that of sprain or strain. Rheumatism and arthritis also involve the joint, and pain may be referred in from other points. How this can be handled is explained here. First, let's spend a moment with sprains and strains.

How to Handle Sprains and Strains via Acupressure, U.S.A.

In addition to the acupuncture points you find indicated in Figure 155, there are certain supplementary procedures to use for better and faster healing.

Physical therapy may consist of compressing the new sprain or strain with the palm of the hand. Apply no more heat than the palm can give. This restrains swelling before you start treatment. It chases out the edema so that you may quickly locate the point of pain. Finger pressure on the "ouch spot" is applied until local pain, muscle spasm, or arterial throbbing has stopped. Massage the muscles *around*, but not over, the lesion. This not only keeps the muscles and tendons pliable, but stimulates circulation and removes collections of lymph waste called "swelling." Immediately pack the ankle in ice. Treatment time a half hour. Apply a laced boot, or wrap with torn sheeting, gauze, or adhesive tape to lock the joint in a figure-eight bandage.

Brief, At-a-Glance Techniques for *ANKLE CONDITIONS*

Procedure: Check your symptoms. Find the acupuncture points . . . acupress!

A B C SCHEDULE OF ACTION

SYMPTOMS	ACUPUNCTURE POINTS TO USE		
	A	B	C
Pain	Sp-7	GB-27	GB-28

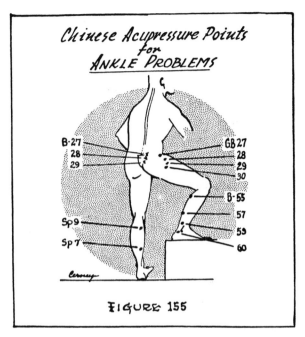

Chinese Acupressure Points
for
ANKLE PROBLEMS

FIGURE 155

Rheumatism	B-59		
Sprain/strain	B-28, 29	B-55, 57 60	GB-27 30
Swelling	Sp-7		

(See preceding Figure 155.)

THE FOOT

For reasons not indicated in Chinese medical history, the sides and top of the human foot are marked by meridians and acupuncture points with only one underneath. Yet, the bottom of the foot reveals a wealth of valuable pressure points, and you have only to probe the bottom of your foot to find them.

I call them *"Z" zones.* They are associate acupuncture points directly related to the nervous systems and the Chinese meridians as well. They are key reflex centers and every foot has them. When there's trouble afoot in the body, these tattletales of deficient health are available for fingertip control. *"Z" zones*, as a vital part of *Acupressure, U.S.A.*, are another way to augment health care by getting to the bottom of it all. In concentrated form, the following chart—on the human foot—gives you 17 different problems affecting the foot and the ABC Schedule of Action in dealing with them. (See also Figure 156.) Following this, you will delve into the amazing power of the *"Z" zones*. (See Figure 23.)

Brief, At-a-Glance Techniques for *FOOT CONDITIONS*

Procedure: Check your condition. Find the acupuncture point . . . acupress!

A B C SCHEDULE OF ACTION

CONDITION	ACUPUNCTURE POINTS TO USE					
	A	**B**	**C**	**D**	**E**	**F**
Aching arch	B-56					
Can't raise foot	Si-9					
Cold feet	Sp-1	Sp-3	Sp-6	K-7	K-26	
Cold and wet feet	K-2					
Cold and paralyzed	Sp-1	Sp-6				
Circulation (poor)	Li-10					
Cramps (spasms)	St-30	St-33	Sp-5	B-23	B-28	B-29 50
Gout	Liv-3	Liv-4	Sp-5	St-43		
Heavy feeling	B-56					
Hot feet	K-1					
Heel pain and swelling	K-5	K-6				

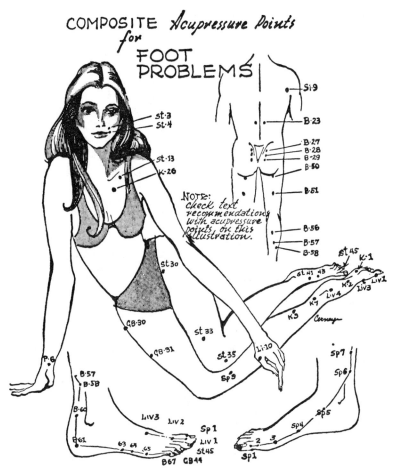

COMPOSITE *Acupressure Points* *for* FOOT PROBLEMS

NOTE: check text recommendations with acupressure points on this illustration.

FIGURE 156

Pain (general)	B-62	K-2	K-9			
Paralysis	St-30	S-42	B-23	B-51 61	K-7	Sp-1, 6
Perspiration (excessive)	St-13					
Rheumatism	St-35	St-41	P-6	B-60		
Swelling	St-3, 4 33, 35	Sp-4 7, 9	K-2	B-27 57, 58	B-62	GB-30 31

Toes (in general)	K-1					
second and 3rd	St-45					
big toe	Liv-1	Sp-1				
4th toe	G-44					
5th toe	B-67					

THE ASTONISHING POWER OF
THE "Z" ZONES
AND HOW TO CONTROL THEM!

Let's take a look at those tattletale points in the human foot that—like Chinese acupuncture points—are trigger points of pain when the body's organs and parts, with which they are intimately associated by nerve, blood, and lymph systems, are not functioning at par. Let's see how *your* foot becomes a sophisticated diagnostic instrument for pointing out that there's physiological trouble afoot, another method in *Acupressure, U.S.A.* that puts you in control.

How are *your* "Z" zones today? Have you checked those warning signals, those press agents that herald the fact that a foot or body problem is in progress, that these "magic buttons"—along with the traditional acupuncture points—can give you instant self-help?

You don't believe it? The fact is, in the beginning, I didn't either. In fact, in my ignorance on the matter, I scoffed. Then I learned that there *is* a health warning system in the human foot! I learned that there *are* more reflex areas than the traditional Chinese doctor outlined. To check this out for yourself, take off your shoes and stockings. Cross one leg over the other. With the bottom of one foot peeking up at you, make an excursion with your thumb down the arch of your foot. With your thumb tip making tiny rotary motions, investigate from end to end. Press!

Find any sore spots? Didn't even know they were there? If your foot does *not* have any of these points of pain, then three points are in order: (1) *you were NOT probing deeply enough*, (2) *you are in remarkably good foot and body health*, or (3) *you're kidding yourself.*

Remember that these reflex points may be just that, pinpoints! As you become more adept at finding them, it will be easier to control your own state of health. Go back and do it again. If, like the rotund English writer, Samuel Johnson, you can't reach your feet, have someone else do it. Get to the bottom of the matter. Ask a friend. Does sudden knowledge of these "sore spots" disturb you? They should. Nature has just told you something! Nature, through those trigger zones in your foot, has just informed you as to the state of health of a given organ or part which that tender "Z" zone represents! This warning signal does not diagnose the problem. It tells you only where the problem is. Very precisely, it tells you that when you are investigating the "Z" zones of your left foot, you are investigating the condition of organs and parts on the left side of your body and head. When you are investigating the right foot, you are pointing out conditions on the right side. Through the amazing network of the blood, nerve, lymph, and Chinese meridian systems, all parts are interconnected.

Study Figure 23. Note how cunningly Nature has arranged each "Z" zone positionally. Even better, note how acupuncture "Z" zones give you fingertip control . . . one of the best things that can happen to you . . . as you treat yourself to health through *acupuncture without needles! Acupressure, U.S.A.!*

"Z" Zones . . . Key Zones to Future Health

"Z" zones, or reflex reaction areas, have no one common or single degree of pain. In accordance with the degree of sensitivity of the person and the duration and the physical problem involved, a "Z" zone manifests itself. Some people experience little or no pain when the "Z" zone is pressed. Others jump. Yet, the same "Z" zones exist in everyone—and when you pinpoint this area, you are not just locating the probable area of non-health, you are using these key zones to restore health. Each zone is not just a warning signal but a center of treatment. In using your "Z" zones, you are not just alleviating local distress, you are re-establishing tone in the organ or part associated with it. You are increasing vitality and causing the various body systems to be more efficient. Toxic waste is released as these systems recuperate, and quite often this accounts for the distress that may be noted after treatment. Release of waste in the body may make you "feel bad." Expect it. If you have triggered the right buttons, Nature will help you by doing the rest. So pinpoint your "Z" zones. Then treat them the same as all other acupuncture points because they are one and the same!

A Housewife Is Rid of Pain
... "For the First Time in Years"

Laura Jean had been medically indoctrinated all the years of her life. Her father was a physician, her mother a former nurse. Laura truly believed that drugs and surgery were the only answer to human problems, that everything else was quackery. She believed this sincerely until two feet of her large intestine was removed because of the pain in her belly. The pain continued. Then came the cutting of nerves or sympathectomy. The pain still continued. The gamut of drugs was run. The pain continued, and that's when her husband disrupted her indoctrination. He was angry that Laura had been subjected to all the surgery and that now they even wanted to remove her ovaries and uterus. He felt there had to be yet another method to try. There was—*Acupuncture ... Without Needles.* Three weeks after initial treatment, Laura sent me a note from their vacation hotel at Miami Beach. "This is the first time in all these years," she wrote, "that I've been free of pain. I use your 'Z' zones every day. Come to think of it, this isn't just a vacation. I feel so good it's like a second honeymoon!"

Index